how cancer improved my life

how cancer improved my life

A JOURNEY OF STRENGTH, COURAGE, AND HOPE WITH A PINCH OF HUMOR, WHILE BATTLING CANCER

CHRISTINE R. SCHRADER

WITH

JANICE JAMES-TOBISCH

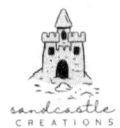

sandcastle
CREATIONS

Library of Congress Control Number: 2025921294

Paperback ISBN: 979-8-9932083- 0-5
Hardback ISBN: 979-8-9932083-1-2
Digital Book ISBN: 979-8-9932083-2-9
Audiobook ISBN: 979-8-9932083-3-6

Pinted in the USA

"People build sandcastles every day... They do it for the day, because we're here now, and because in this moment it shows that these are the things that matter to us"

— ROBERT J. CRANE - AUTHOR

contents

2015

2016

foreword

BY GAYLE FLAIG

Writing this foreword about Christine is both a joy and an honor. I had the privilege of working as one of her supervisors at Genesis Child Development Center, part of Regis Catholic Schools. She started at the center in September 2013. During her illness, we grew to have a special friendship. I will always cherish the conversations we shared, and the moments of trust we built - even accompanying her to the emergency room a few times when she needed support. Those experiences deepened my admiration for her courage, her strength, and her grace. I came to know her not just as a wonderful teacher, but as an extraordinary person.

It seems only fitting that Christine chose to work within the Catholic school system, since she herself attended both Immaculate Conception Elementary School and Regis High School. Having grown up within this community, it was wonderful for her to give back to children with the same dedication and faith-filled spirit that shaped her own childhood. Her journey reflects a beautiful full circle - one that enriched both her life and the lives of the children she worked with.

Christine was a gifted teacher who touched countless lives with her kindness, patience, and creativity. Children loved her for the way she made them feel special and safe, while parents deeply valued the trust and care she provided. She helped shape numerous little lives, creating memories and lessons that will stay with them forever.

What stands out about Christine is not just her devotion to the children, but also the way she gave of herself in every setting. Her talents extended beyond the classroom. Christine loved volunteering for center events, whether it was creating the table decor for the family harvest breakfast, or managing the Scholastic book fair, she was always willing to help. And if the toy storage or art storage closets needed organizing, Christine was the go-to person. As a co-worker, she was known for her strong work ethic and her generosity of spirit. Her presence enriched our team.

This book is a testament to the difference one person can make in the lives of so many. Christine's story is one of celebration, faith, and genuine care for others. Her life is a reflection of her values, reminding us that when faith and service come together, the result is a life that inspires and uplifts all who were blessed to know her.

Gayle Flaig
Administrator of Early Childhood Programs
Regis Catholic Schools

letter to the reader

Dear Reader,

It has taken some time to complete this book. Grief is like a slippery eel, you think you have a good hold on it and then it rears up it's head and flips you on your back!

Christine was a very organized young woman. She always had a project or even more in progress. It was as if she didn't want to miss a single thing. She lived a full life not wanting to miss a moment in it. Christine highly valued her friendships. She was extremely loyal and she expected no less from those close to her.

When Christine was diagnosed with cancer, she took it on like it was the biggest project of her life. She rallied her sisters, two who are nurses, medical personnel and friends. She set up a blog on CaringBridge to keep contact with loved ones while allowing herself to process what she had to deal with that day. In her entries we find her project for a book and what she wanted it to accomplish. Even with the ups and downs of treatment, she wanted to give help and hope to others. Her entries have been left as she wrote them.

Treatment was intense and long. She had over sixty rounds of chemo in the four years of fighting the cancer. Her fight for life was also intense, as was her need to have it not be in vain. In her final hours she had family giving comfort and company during another intense time.

"I will get the book done for you..." and "I love you." With her reply, "I love you too," which were her last words.

This is Christine's GIFT to all who find themselves lost in a world of emotions dealing with horrible news about their health or a loved ones health. May this book give hope and to accomplish why it was written.

She believed she could and fought to her last breath trying.

She is so loved and is missed very much.

Janice James-Tobisch

2014

hello friends and family!

I am very new to all this, so please bear with me.

Two weeks ago, I went to the doctor for a colonoscopy. Having had issues with my digestion for many months, this was the procedure that was needed to determine whether I had IBS, IBD (irritable bowel disease), or something else. After the procedure, the doctor had informed me that a mass had been found and that he had taken a biopsy of the mass and would have the results in the next few days. I went to work as usual the next two days, and on Wednesday, August 20th; while at work, I was given the very unfortunate news that the mass they had found was cancerous.

I was floored! My world had just been completely flipped upside down, and I had no idea what to do. The director at my work is more than amazing and let me leave work early that day—immediately after I got the news, actually. In her office, I completely broke down and told her everything that was going on.

On my way home, I received a call from the administrator of the Child Development Center I work at (she's the top boss :)). She was so supportive and made sure that I knew they were all there for me. I started to feel a bit better after talking to them. I had already started to form a support team, and I hadn't even told my family yet.

Once I got home, I called my sister, Sue Ann (the one in Chicago). We talked for over an hour, and I could feel the hope start to build in my body. Yeah, I got horrible news today, but I am going to beat this. My sister had called my mom and two other sisters to let them know what was going on. I immediately began receiving texts letting me know that when I was ready to talk, they were there for me. My little sister told my dad, and he was just as supportive as everyone else... and yet again, my support team was growing.

Later that day, I was called by the hospital to start setting up doctors' appointments. I was scheduled to have a CT scan the following day (to see if it had spread anywhere else), an appointment with oncology and surgery the following Tuesday. Now it was starting to get a bit overwhelming. That night, when I went to bed, I prayed the rosary and asked God to give me the strength to get through tomorrow. This may sound like something little to ask for when I could be asking to be cured, but whatever happens down the road, it's still a day-to-day process. It wasn't as overwhelming when I thought to myself, "It doesn't matter what happens next week, next month, or next year, you just need to get through today!"

I had my CT scan but had to wait until the following Tuesday to get the results. I just continued to pray and asked God for the strength to get through the following day. Sue Ann came up on Monday night so that she was able to go to my doctor's appointments with me. Tuesday morning, we met with the oncologist, and he informed me that they had found masses in my lungs, liver, and lymph nodes. Now I had to have another scan called a PET scan (positron emission tomography scan) to determine whether these masses were cancerous as well. If they were, I would need to have another CT scan (also known as a CAT scan—computerized tomography scan), at which time they would biopsy one of the masses to determine the makeup of the cancer profile. I was oddly calm after this appointment and even went back to work for a few hours. Later that day, I had my surgery consult, and after meeting with the surgeon. He had determined that because there was a good chance the cancer had spread; he didn't want to do surgery yet. "I don't want to do surgery because it will not cure you," were his actual words. I felt as if my "Hope Balloon" had just been popped. I once again broke down, feeling completely overwhelmed and defeated. I had to go back to work to get my car, and I once again talked to the amazing ladies I work for.

Let me just add a quick side note here that states the type of cancer that I have been currently diagnosed with (colorectal cancer) is EXTREMELY rare in someone my age. And after talking with the girls at work, I began to think about the news I had received that day. Neither my oncologist nor general surgeon has EVER seen this type of case in someone my age. That means there are no statistics to go off of. No one but God knows how this book is going to end! I have been urged to go see some specialists down in Rochester, and I have already started to put that in the works.

My PET scan on Wednesday has shown that the masses are cancerous and will need to be biopsied (which I was expecting) and has been scheduled for this week.

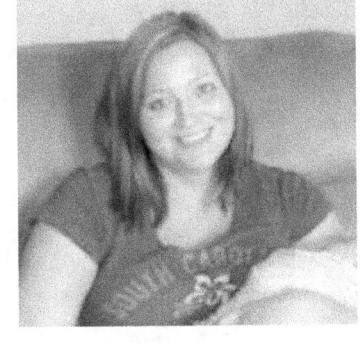

Wow! What a couple of weeks, huh? It has been a whirlwind, and some days are better than others, but what I need is the love and support from all my family and friends. My daily goal is to stay positive, to live it to the fullest, and to get through it... whatever it entails.

Some of you may know this, but my motto has always been, "Dance like you do when no one is watching. Love like you've never been hurt. And live like there's no tomorrow."

It definitely takes on a new meaning now, and even though I have had it as my motto for well over ten years, I finally understand it today!

Love to you all!

All my Love,
Christine

i can feel the love

Thank you all for all the well-wishes and support!

The amount of love and care I have seen is truly inspiring. I hope everyone had a great Labor Day. I had a really good day yesterday. Being able to read all the comments and guest book entries filled me with even more hope that I am going to "Fight It Like A Beast!" (If you haven't caught on yet, this is our saying for kicking cancer's butt. :) Thank you, Sarah!)

It was nice to have a day filled with laughter instead of talking about upcoming biopsies and such! I had lunch with my bestie Kate and her adorable son Crosby—and then I hung out with my sisters (Sue Ann and Sarah) for the rest of the day.

We went through some old family photos (Sarah assures me I have blackmail on 90% of the Schrader family... watch out on Throwback Thursdays. Haha), and then we had a Guac-Off. Each of us made guacamole, and my boyfriend Dan chose the winner through a blind taste test. And wouldn't you know, Sarah (the one who has never made it before) won! Now it's back to work and preparing for my biopsy on

Thursday. I will keep you all posted here. Thank you for keeping me in your prayers!

All my Love,
Christine

"one small positive thought in the morning can change your entire day."

SEPT. 4, 2014, 6:21 PM

What a day it's been!

I started off today with my biopsy consult with Dr. Jean Baptiste (I took this as a very good sign, as his name is super close to John the Baptist—Haha). When he entered the exam room, he gave me a very confused look, walked out, and then walked back in. I told him my name, and he said, "Oh! So, I am in the right room. I'm just used to seeing much older patients."

Yep, I've heard that a lot over the last two weeks. I think my body believes it's older than it is. He went over the procedure, the risks, and all that info. I didn't learn any new info pertaining to the initial diagnosis; however, they are doing the biopsy to do genetic testing, and to make sure they know where it started from. They will be doing a biopsy of my right lung, and with the information obtained, they will be able to say for sure if it's colorectal cancer that has spread to my lungs or vice versa.

The lung biopsy has been scheduled for next Tuesday, the 9th. I will be sedated for this procedure, so I'm not sure how soon I will be able to update everyone, but Sue Ann is an author on my page, so you may get an update from her.

After the doctor, I went back to work and worked the rest of the day. Man, those babies meant business today! Haha. They took no prisoners!!! I am truly looking forward to tomorrow. TGIF!!

I have been asked numerous times over the last two weeks, "You are taking this really well, how can you stay positive?" And the answer is... that is my only option—to stay positive. Each morning, I get up and thank God for giving me another day to fight this like a beast, and every night, I ask him for the strength to get through tomorrow. And then He sends me your amazing messages, and texts, and phone calls. I cherish each and every one! So, I guess another way to answer that question is that I stay positive because I have so many loving friends and family telling me I can beat this, and I BELIEVE THEM!

All my love, and... GO PACK GO!

All my Love,
Christine

done with the biopsy

SEPT. 9, 2014, 11:10 AM

I just got out of my lung biopsy, and everything went great! They are watching me for the next few hours (which is standard) to make sure there are no complications. But the doctor said everything went as planned. We won't get the results for a few days, but I will keep you posted. Thanks again for your love and support!

All my Love,
Christine

be positive... it's not only my mantra; it's my blood type!

SEPT. 13, 2014, 10:30 AM

Yesterday was a looooooong day!

I had gotten a voicemail on Thursday saying that I had missed my doctor's appointment with Dr. C, my oncologist, and needed to reschedule. This was news to me as I was never informed of the appointment. I was able to reschedule it for Friday (yesterday), and the amazing ladies at work were once again able to get me out of work so I could go.

Dan (my boyfriend) took a half day from work to go with me as Sue Ann had already headed back to Chicago. I was extremely nervous for the appointment, but I had a feeling I knew what news he was going to give me. The night before, I had asked God for a double dose of strength as I was going to need it to get through the day. "Ask and you shall receive." We talked to the doctor, and he informed me that the biopsy had shown that it was colorectal cancer that had spread to my lungs, liver, and lymph nodes. Dan says I'm lucky I don't have any other body parts that start with an "L." Haha.

Because it has spread to multiple places, it is considered stage 4, but my doctor is hopeful that he can control it and put it into remission! I had to ask exactly what remission meant, and this is what he told me: if you were to take another CT scan, you would still see the tumors, but they are not growing or causing any issues... basically dormant. The chances of total remission are 10% in which I told him, "Doc, I'm a pretty rare person... You'd better recheck your numbers." He chuckled and agreed with me.

So, now for the treatment plan. Right now (and this may change), the plan is to get my port implanted on Wednesday. A port is a surgical implant that will allow them to start IVs, do blood draws, and do chemo without having to find a vein (which I am very excited about... feeling a bit like a pincushion these days). On Thursday, I will start chemo, and from what I understood, I will be hooked up to a portable pump and then sent home for two days, at which time, I will go back to the hospital, and they will remove the pump. So, I will be having chemo at home. I asked the doctor how soon until my hair falls out, and he told me that it would thin out a bit, but I would not be completely bald. Hallelujah! As soon as I knew chemo was an option, I began preparing myself to lose all my hair and thought of the options: wig, hats, Mr. Clean. As I thought about it, a wig wasn't a realistic option for work. I could just imagine the first time a child pulled it off my head and realized it could come off... now we just started a game. Haha. I would never be able to sit on the floor again; they would constantly be trying to snatch my wig off! So that is the game plan so far. Every two weeks, I will have a chemo treatment, and we will do four rounds. At the end of the four rounds, it will be reassessed, and a new plan will be made.

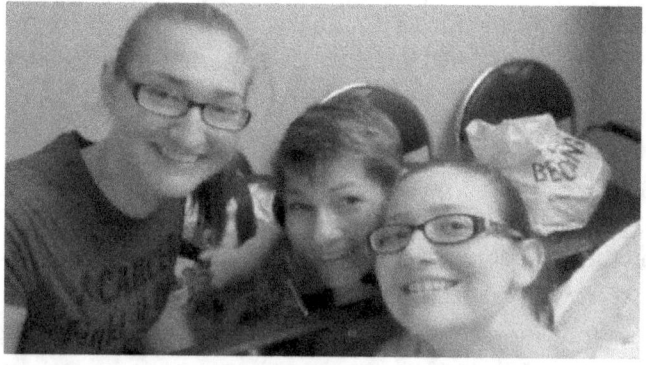

Day by day!

Now for some inspiration...

Many people have told me how angry they feel that this happened to me. They don't understand why bad things happen to good people, and they ask me if I feel the same. I don't. I'm not mad at God that I got sick. I'm not angry that I try to lead a good life, and I have been given this huge obstacle. When we ask God for something (patience, love, understanding, etc.), He just doesn't give it to us; He gives us tasks that require us to build what we asked for. He gives us opportunities to be patient, to love someone when it's hard, and to understand the way someone else is feeling. So please, if you are feeling anger or frustration with God over what has happened to me, or anyone for that matter, know that through him I will "Fight This Like A Beast." Take a deep breath, think of me, and let it go. POSITIVITY!

All my Love,
Christine

a port on the starboard side

SEPT. 17, 2014, 8:05 PM

What a day! I feel like my days are getting longer and longer. Today was the day I got my port implanted in my chest. Thank you, Jesus!!!! No more feeling like a pincushion, multiple sticks per week, or bruises! The surgery went great, and there were no complications at all. I have been told I was pretty funny coming off the sedation,

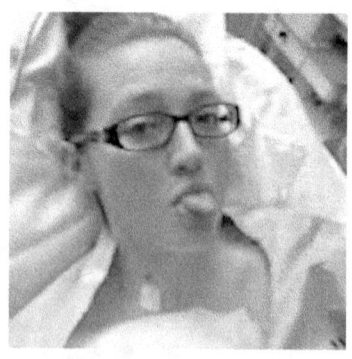

and thank goodness, there were no video cameras present at this time. Haha. After a few hours in recovery, I was discharged and ran a few errands before heading home. Now I am resting comfortably at home (I was sent home with more Vicodin) very comfortably and have Sarah and Sue Ann waiting on me hand and foot. I could get used to this! :)

Well, just a quick update tonight, and now it's time for bed. Tomorrow, I start chemo, and I will post again to keep you all in the loop. Thank you again for all your love and positive thoughts!

All my Love,
Christine

a recipe for success!

SEPT. 18, 2014, 10:13 PM

Yesterday was the day... the day I started chemotherapy. I was pretty nervous going into the appointment because I wasn't sure what side effects I was going to have. Flashbacks from the movie *Dying Young*, with Julia Roberts, kept flooding my mind. First, I had a blood draw out of my BRAND SPANKING NEW PORT, and it went amazingly. No pain, no digging with needles. It was quick and painless. When they put in my port, they had placed the needle so they wouldn't need to poke a brand-new port. If you look at the "awesome" picture Sue Ann attached to the last update, you can kind of make out a large stack of gauze piled on my chest. I actually looked like I had half a boob job done instead of a port implanted. Haha. The amazing tech at the cancer center took out the original needle that was a good inch off my chest and switched it out with a low-profile needle that only lies less than a half inch off my chest.

I then had a meeting with Dr. C, and he went over the side effects to expect for my first treatment. For the first day, he was pretty sure I was only going to be tired. I was to be given steroids prior to treatment to help combat the nausea and sent home with anti-nausea medication to keep it at bay at home. He said it was very rare to have moderate nausea the day of treatment. There's that word again... "rare." Yep, I ended up getting sick before I left the hospital. I'm thinking I need to change my middle name to Rare. That way, my initials are still the same. How my treatments will work is that every other Thursday, I will be getting half of my treatment at the cancer center, and then I will go home with a pump that contains the rest of the treatment, and I will be wearing this for the next two days.

Before I even started my treatment, Sue Ann and I sported awesome stick-on mustaches and quickly became the talk of the cancer center. Lots of giggles, thumbs-ups, and smiles passed my doorway. Laughter is the best medicine. The wonderful ladies gave me a gift because it was my first day. I was given a prayer shawl made by a woman from Pigeon Falls, WI. It is absolutely beautiful, and I was happy to receive it!

The symptoms I had yesterday were nausea (bad enough to lose all my lunch), fatigue, and an increase in the sensitivity to cold in my hands and feet, which should only last a few days. I spent the rest of the night on the couch, sipping tea and going in and out of sleep. I took some anti-nausea medicine before bed and slept fairly well. I did, however, get up and 2:00 am and couldn't get back to sleep until 4:00. This morning, I am feeling pretty good. I had some eggs and tea for breakfast and took some more steroids to help with the nausea and fatigue.

I have a cardiology appointment that is just a routine yearly visit this morning. With how well I am feeling right now, we are going to run some errands and be back in time for a nap! Love my naps!!!

I hope everyone enjoys their day and gets to experience the beautiful day we are going to have.

All my Love,
Christine

take that, cancer!

SEPT. 21, 2014, 3:56 PM

S unday Funday is here! It's amazing how different it is now. After going to church, I went to the farmers' market to get some yummy veggies for BLTs today. I have somehow developed a milk sensitivity to all dairy products, so I have to pretty much make everything myself to ensure there is no dairy in any of my food. If you live in Wisconsin, it should be IMPOSSIBLE for a person to have a milk allergy or sensitivity. I'm not gonna lie... it blows! But a bonus is that I can start eating clean, which is really good for keeping my body healthy. Eating clean consists of taking a lot of processed food out of your diet and using only fresh vegetables, fruits, and proteins. So today, Dan and I had BLTs with turkey bacon, lettuce, and tomatoes—fresh from the farmers' market. It was one of the best BLTs I have ever had.

The Princess Bride was on TV, so I watched the end of that and then took a nap. I missed the Packers' game, but it sounds like I didn't miss much. Haha. We have a low-key afternoon planned and pork fajitas for dinner. YUM!

This weekend went great as it was my first "Chemo Weekend." My doctor has me taking steroids each morning and two different anti-nausea medications to combat the nausea, which I hardly had to take this weekend—they are an as-needed medication. I am on my chemo pump to combat the fatigue. I still did need to take some naps throughout the day; usually, a thirty-minute catnap would do, and I was ready for the day. The only other side effect I had this weekend was an increased sensitivity to cold. Reaching into the fridge or freezer makes my hand feel like I just touched a metal pole in 30-below-zero weather. Sue Ann and I went to Orange Leaf (a frozen yogurt shop in Eau Claire), and they had dairy-free sorbet! I have not had ice cream in months, so I jumped at the fact that I could have an ice cream substitute. I got a sample, and with the first bite, I felt the feeling of sticking my tongue to a metal pole in the middle of winter. Oh yeah! I have an increased sensitivity to cold. I didn't let that stop me! I just ate it really, really slowly, and it was amazing! Haha. The side effect has and will lessen as the chemo drugs are filtered out of my system. So, I will soon be able to drink beverages above room temperature.

I was expecting to be in bed all weekend, and I was so grateful and happy to be able to enjoy the weekend with my sisters. I am off the chemo pump for eleven days, and then I go back for round two of four. Positive thoughts that the next round will go even better than the last.

Thank you for all your well-wishes and supportive comments on here, in person, and in emails/texts. They are so helpful and motivating to me. I enjoy reading them and sharing them with friends and family. So... please keep them coming.

All my Love,
Christine

the struggle you are in today, is developing the strength you need for tomorrow!

Wow! I can't believe a whole week has already gone by. It was really weird to work all week with no doctor's appointments to go to. By Friday, I was tired! This week has gone really well. I have had a lot of energy, and my appetite has been really good (I ate half a rotisserie chicken by myself on Monday as well as sweet corn). Not too much happened this week. I worked, and that was about it. This weekend, I canned pickles, salsa, and dilly beans (pickled green beans) with my dad on Saturday. We ended with seven jars of salsa, seven jars of pickles, and four jars of dilly beans. My dad informed me that this apparently isn't a lot. When he cans, he usually has double digits of the number of cans. I see why it is usually a whole-weekend ordeal.

After our canning experience, I was invited over for dinner at my grandma's house for tacos!! Love me some tacos! A few of my aunts were over as well, and I was able to visit with them for a while. My Aunt Julie brought me an "I'm sorry you have cancer" gift. She found an awesome gift called a "Dammit Doll." I will try to attach a picture of it because it is a little hard to explain, but I love it! She also made me a T-shirt in Hayward that reads, "Stay Strong." And I will!!! While talking with my family, I discovered that my grandma and aunt have a dairy sensitivity as well. We swapped dairy substitutes, and I even got to try soy cheese. It's not as bad as you would think, as long as it's cold.

Today, I went to church in the morning and then hit up the farmers' market for some veggies for the week. This has become my weekly ritual, and I am going to be sad when it's done for the season. I was able to find dairy-free bread and bagels at the festival, and I had some amazing tomatoes from my Aunt Julie, so I had BLTs again today. Haha. They are just so good! This time, I made them with real bacon, and they were even better than before.

For the rest of the day, I didn't do too much. I had a sewing project I was working on, and Dan and I watched the movie "Draft Day." I really enjoyed the movie even though I had no idea how the NFL Draft worked. I had to ask a few questions during the movie, but I don't think Dan minded. Haha.

This coming week is going to be a lot busier. I work Monday through Wednesday. I have chemo on Thursday, and my mom and oldest sister, Jenny, will be coming up. As long as I tolerate it as well as the last time, we have some fun things planned, including staying overnight in the cities. I am so excited as I have not seen my sister, Jenny, in almost two years.

I will get my blood tested on Thursday, and that info will tell us how my body is reacting to the chemo. My iron level has gone up two points and is only two more points from normal, which is why I have had so much more energy. They will be able to tell how much my red and/or white blood cell count has gone down since my first round of chemotherapy, if any.

My increased sensitivity to cold is gone but will come back on Thursday... I better go eat some sorbet before then!

All in all, it was a very normal week, which I thoroughly enjoyed! Thank you to all those who are praying and supporting me through this. You may be praying for me, but I am praying for you. I thank God every day for having you all in my life and to bless you all for caring enough to send me your positive thoughts and love! I truly could not have done this without you!

All my Love,
    Christine

"i don't know if you know this, but we are kinda a big deal."

OCT. 3, 2014, 6:53 PM

Round two of chemo is in full swing. All the nurses were excited to see Sarah and me in our very stylish mustaches. I made sure to eat breakfast and even had a snack before chemo started, and I still got nauseous, but it wasn't bad enough to make me "toss my cookies!" I took a nap, which Sarah so lovely took pictures of and put on Facebook... she better be ready for the repercussions of that. Watch Facebook for the pictures I have of her. Haha.

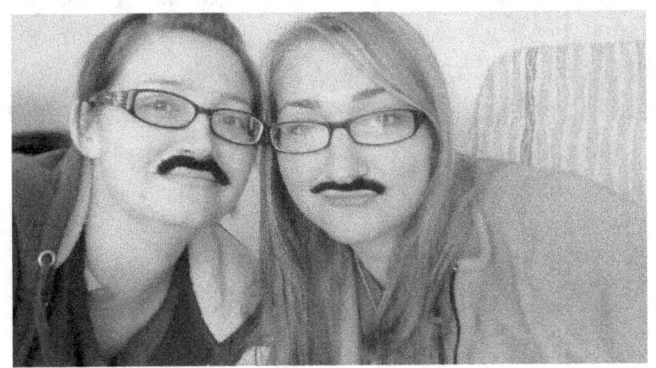

The nausea lasted most of the night, and I wasn't able to eat anything until about 9:00 pm, which consisted of oyster crackers and warm Powerade. With the steroids I'm on, my sleep schedule is all screwed up. I was up from about midnight until 4:00 am. My mom and oldest sister, Jenny from Colorado, both came into town last night, but my sister didn't fly into the cities until 10:00 pm, so I didn't get to see her until today.

Today, my mom and sister came over around 11:30 this morning. We ran to Buffalo Wild Wings for lunch, yet another place I have found with a dairy-free menu! They tasted soooo good! Once we stuffed ourselves with fries and wings, we ran over to my mom's old boss's house to have some pictures reprinted. She used to work at a photography studio, and he now runs it out of his house. He's going to look for my cap and gown picture from high school graduation, as the only picture I have is on my graduation announcement. After a quick run to Target, we went to the mall to get some new shoes, and gloves, and scarves for the non-Wisconsinites who thought it was "SO COLD" out today. My brother, Ken, came over tonight to make me BBQ chicken for dinner, which is the best chicken I have ever had. My appetite has been pretty good today, but it has been hard to drink water as I can't be colder than room temperature due to my cold sensitivity. My weight has stayed the same as the last time I went into chemo, which is really good that I have been able to maintain it for two weeks.

My doctor is very happy with the results after the first round of chemo and is extremely hopeful for the second round. He believes that by the time I'm done with the second round that all the symptoms I have been having from the masses will be gone! Which is awesome news!! My red blood cell, white blood cell, and platelet levels are all in the normal range, which is awesome. The prayers and positive thoughts are definitely helping, so please keep them coming. Here's to a great weekend with family, and I hope all your weekends

All my Love,
      Christine

girls just wanna have fun

OCT. 6, 2014, 7:53 PM

Round two of chemo is officially over, and we celebrated by having a girl's weekend in the Twin Cities. My sisters, Jenny and Sarah, my mom, and I went up after my chemo pump came off to spend the night and do a little shopping. We didn't have a lot of time, but we had fun in the time we had. We went to the Mall of America on Saturday night and did some shopping and had dinner. Once we got back to the hotel, we did facials and had some popcorn. It was like a little sleepover with some of my favorite people! Jenny had to fly out really early in the morning on Sunday, so Sarah and I drove her to the airport and sent her off. My mom had an eleven-hour drive to make on Sunday, too; so, we figured she needed as much sleep as she could get. She left around 7:00, and Sarah and I promptly went back to sleep. Haha. We took advantage of the noon checkout by sleeping as long as we could. It wasn't until 10:00 am that hunger won over and I took Sarah on her first trip to Denny's. Even though I looked up what was dairy-free at the restaurant and informed the waiter of my dairy allergy, milk still made its way into my meal. Sarah and I packed up the hotel and went to a few more stores, including Ikea. It was about now that I realized there was milk in my breakfast, and we decided to head home. Even after sleeping a good chunk of the morning, Sarah and I were tired.

By the time I got home, it was already 3:30, so I set my bags by the door and crawled right into bed for a nap. It wasn't until 5:00 pm that I woke up. The rest of the night was pretty low-key. I watched the movie *Blended*, and loved it! I recommend it, especially if you like *Wedding Singer* or *50 First Dates*. This morning was tough to get out of bed, but I think it was more of the fact that it was so cold and that it was still dark out.

Work went really well today. It went really fast, and I even got to leave a little early. With my treatment plan and the very good possibility of surgery before the end of the year, I will be switching from an infant teacher to a float teacher. I do love my babies, but with the chances of my treatment plan changing, this will give them the consistency they need. I could be out of work for up to six weeks after surgery, so having someone already trained in that position will make it a lot easier. My end goal is that once surgery is over and my schedule is more consistent, I will be able to be transitioned back into my infant room. I absolutely love working with children of that age, and my co-teacher is amazing! Miss Cassie is the best co-teacher in the world, and we work so well together. Also, with being a float teacher, it will make my schedule more flexible for doctor's visits and if I need some extra time off. Everyone at work has been so great, and the parents have been giving me encourage-ment and well-wishes. I truly work at the best child care center ever!

Just like the previous round of chemo, my body has been responding really well. I have little fatigue, my appetite has been good (I ate three rolls of sushi, which is about eighteen pieces, for dinner tonight with Sarah), and there has been no nausea. God has definitely given me the tools I need to beat this horrible disease. He has given me the strength to get through each day, the love and support of family and friends, and the knowledge of a great doctor who has customized my treatment plan to make it bearable for me to get through each round. Thank you for your continued support and love.

All my Love,
Christine

why you gotta be so sassy?

OCT. 11, 2014, 9:43 AM

Another week has flown by! But it feels like way more time has passed since my mom and sister were up last weekend. Round two of chemo went great, and I have even fewer symptoms and side effects now. My cold sensitivity hung around longer this time, but it was mostly in my hands, and I think it was due to the fact that it is unbelievably cold outside most of the day. I definitely needed mittens on my way out the door each morning. I feel more energized and have been getting better sleep at night. My body is reacting extremely well to treatment, and I know it has to do with all the prayers and positive thoughts I have been getting from all of you!

On Thursday, I will start my third treatment out of four and will hopefully be getting another scan in the first part of November. Depending on how the scan looks, I could be looking at more chemo, radiation, or surgery. It's a little up in the air, but I just take it day by day and thank God for giving me today to fight this... like a beast!

After talking with people about my journey, I sometimes get, "You're really doing good, right? You're not just putting on a show and then crying when no one's around." Let me assure all of you that I am being 100% honest in person, on my page, and all throughout the day. I'm not saying that I don't have my down days when it gets a little over-whelming or I think too much of what the future may or may not bring, but I choose to have lots more good days than bad. I know that I could die from this, but I am not going to focus on that. I will prepare for the different outcomes, but I will put my love, strength, and stub-bornness behind beating this! I was told that one in three women will get some form of cancer in their lives. Now, granted, I'm not sure how accurate this statistic is, and if you have been reading my posts, you know how much I love proving statistics wrong. But when I got to thinking about that statistic, if I have a one in three chance that I could get cancer, I would rather fight it when I am young, healthy, and super sassy! I think this journey would be a lot harder if I were married, had children, and were unable to tolerate the chemo as well. I'm not saying I'm glad I have. Cancer, but I am glad that I have a higher chance of beating this! Last week, Sarah, the baby sister, was asking about a previous post where I had mentioned that God doesn't always give us what we want, but he gives us opportunities. She paused for a moment and asked me, "Did you ask God if you wanted to be skinny a lot?" Now, I couldn't help but laugh because Sarah has questions or comments like this all the time. No, I don't think God gave me cancer because I wanted to be skinny. I guess I never think of it as God giving me cancer for any reason. But it was her next comment that really made me laugh. She said, "Because I asked God to help me get in shape, and now I have to bike seven miles to work." Moral of Sarah's story: be careful what you pray for! Haha.

Have a great weekend and enjoy the beautiful fall weather we are having! Something definitely needs to be made in the crockpot this weekend!

All my Love,
Christine

staching up!

OCT. 17, 2014, 8:12 AM

Round three started even better than the last two. I did get nauseous yesterday, but it didn't last as long and wasn't as severe as before. The doctor gave me an extra dose of Ativan before I left for nausea, which made me sleep from 4:00 pm to 7:00 am, on and off. I was only actually up for about three to four hours.

The cold sensitivity is a little worse than before, but that might just be because the weather is a lot cooler than before. I'm back to drinking a lot of herbal tea and warmed-up Powerade. Sounds gross, I know. So far, no nausea today, and I'm feeling very energized after my twelve hours of sleep last night. I am planning on heading to Milwaukee today to help my sister, Sue Ann, out with the girls. She is making her amazing macaroons for her friend's book release party tonight, and with her husband on drill this weekend, she needed someone to watch the girls. I will take any opportunity to see my nieces, so I was glad to help out, especially after all she has done for me! I'm still astonished at all the gifts and cards that I get every week. Yesterday I received some gifts from one of my chemo nurses. She had found a mustache keychain and a mustache picture frame. I love all my nurses and doctors at Mayo!

Many people have asked about giving donations toward my medical bills, and I have to admit that it makes me a little uncomfortable asking for money for myself. After a lot of consideration, I have set up a page on GoFundMe (https://www.gofundme.com/fy720w). CaringBridge will still be my main form of informing everyone about what's going on in my life.

My cold sensitivity is acting up now with all this typing and causes my hands to cramp up, so this will be a short entry, but I will definitely make another entry this weekend!

All my love,
Christine

life isn't about waiting for the storm to pass; it's learning to dance in the rain

OCT. 23, 2014, 7:55 AM

What a gloomy day! I was thankful I got to sleep in this morning, as I do not have to work until eleven this morning, so I get to relax a bit before work. I love staying snuggled in bed while listening to the rain outside. I have been sleeping so well and even sleeping through the night. Before I started chemo, I would get up every night about every two to three hours. So, to be able to sleep seven to eight hours with only getting up once or not at all is a huge victory for me. That may also be one of the reasons I have more energy now than I did before. The doctor also put me on an iron supplement once a day to boost my blood levels.

After the second round of chemo, my white blood cells took a pretty big hit. They are low, but the doctor says they are still pretty close to the "normal" range. He is very excited to hear that my symptoms are gone and that my side effects are limited. After my fourth round of chemo next Thursday, I will be scheduled for another scan. I am going to guess it will be a CT scan, as I cannot do an MRI due to my implants, and a PET scan can only be completed on Wednesdays, as it is a mobile unit.

This scan should be happening in the first part of November, either one to two weeks after chemo. If my body is reacting as well as we think it is, the doctor may do another four rounds of chemo to shrink the masses even more before we go through with surgery. This would mean a less invasive surgery, which could mean less time off of work. Always a good thing!

I cannot believe it is November next week! Where did October go? The trees have changed, and the weather is definitely colder. I am excited to make slow cooker meals and bake. I made sugar cookies for our work's bake sale earlier this week, and while I was icing them, I thought, "How bad would I feel if I just ate one cookie?" Apparently, I have asked God for more self-control A LOT in the past because it took a lot not to eat one of those cookies! Fingers crossed for my milk allergy to be gone by Christmas so I can eat all the yummy cookies and treats of the season.

I just want to say thank you to all those who have sent me cards, gifts, and well-wishes. I really wanted to send thank-you cards to all of you, but I am so behind now, I don't know if I would be able to get them out. I still may try, but I do want you all to know that I am so appreciative of all that you have done. I enjoy reading the cards and opening the packages. I mean, who doesn't love getting mail! God really has outdone himself with the amount of support and love that he has brought into my life!

All my Love,
Christine

untitled

OCT. 31, 2014, 8:26 PM

Round four of four is close to an end, as I will get my pump off tomorrow afternoon. Yesterday, I was nauseous and pretty out of it; a second dose of lorazepam will do that. But I got up this morning and felt really good. I went to work to see all the kids dressed up in their costumes during the Halloween parade. After that, I was able to run some errands and made it back to the house for a well-deserved nap. After my nap, I made dinner and started handing out candy. I think I ate more that I actually handed out. Haha. We didn't have too many, but with how cold and windy it was, it was hard to believe kids stayed out very long.

During my appointment with my doctor, he told me that he wants to schedule a CT scan on Tuesday, the eleventh, and I will get the results on Wednesday, the twelfth. Sue Ann is thinking about coming up for a few days to go to the doctor's appointment with me. I will also be going for a fifth round of chemo on the twelfth and, more than likely, the doctor will be adding on three more rounds for a total of eight rounds. He said in other cases he has seen 80-90% shrinkage of the masses and that in 10% of the cases the tumors will have 100% dissolved. This is the outcome I am praying for. If that is the case, I will be heading into surgery this month to remove the tissue that was infected to ensure it does not grow back.

My doctor, Doctor C, has been great. He has been extremely positive and hopeful about my treatment plan. I have noticed more thinning of my hair, but not enough to see any different and also the cold sensitivity lasts pretty much the whole time now in my fingers and toes. The doctor says that it is most likely because the weather is a lot colder, and if it were during the summer, I probably wouldn't even notice it.

Now, a very positive note. I have had small amounts of dairy over the last three days, and I have had no effect to it! I am so excited to hopefully start adding dairy back into my diet. I will probably continue to substitute a majority of it, butter and milk, but I've got to have my cheese and yogurt! I have missed them so much. Haha. It's amazing how much I can miss certain foods. Bring on the cheese curds! I really don't mind the milk or butter alternatives, but the cheese alternative is not good and is super expensive.

Thank you again for all your prayers and positive thoughts. I know that God is hearing them and that they are working. People have come up to me who don't know I am sick and tell me how great I look and ask me what I am doing. I think them for the compliment and then have the awkward conversation of why I have lost sixty pounds in one year. But God has given me the strength not only to get through those conversations but also the physical strength to tolerate the treatment that will rid the masses from my body. Prayer and positivity are definitely the tools to beat this disease, and you have all delivered more than I could ever ask!

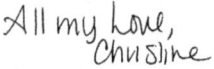

All my Love,
Christine

staching through the snow!

NOV. 11, 2014, 8:35 AM

Today is the day of my CT scan. I am currently drinking the lovely solution needed for my scan... can you sense the sarcasm? Haha. It's not as bad as the prep for a colonoscopy. Please send lots of positive energy and prayers my way. Tomorrow, I will get the results and will post another update to let you know what they are. I'm off of work for the rest of the week after today because chemo was pushed up a day, so I will be going to round five tomorrow. With how cold it is supposed to be over the next week, I'm pretty sure I will be staying indoors as much as I can. Drive safely on this very snowy day!

All my Love,
Christine

he said to her, "daughter, your faith has healed you. go in peace and be freed from your suffering." mark 5:34

This Bible verse was on one of the many get-well cards I received from Regis Middle School students last week. It is a verse I know, hold with me and think about daily. Through God, all things are possible, and if the results from my last CT scan don't show that, I don't know what will!

On Tuesday, I had a CT scan, and by chance, I had the same two nurses from my lung biopsy. While being prepped for the scan, they had recognized me and were excited because they rarely get to know what happens after the procedure or the outcomes of that procedure. I told them that the biopsy did come back as stage four colorectal cancer, and that I had already been on four rounds of chemo. She asked me how it was going, and I let her know that I had little nausea (usually just the day of chemo) and no vomiting, lots of energy, appetite, and I still had my hair. A smile came across her face, and she replied, "Yeah, you look pretty bright-eyed and bushy-tailed today!" The odds of my having both of these nurses for my scan were extremely rare, as they both rarely work together and usually only work with doctors during procedures... God's plan!

Wednesday, Sue Ann, Sarah, and I all went to the doctor's appointment (Sue Ann drove up the night before and came in after midnight... I love my sisters!). We anxiously waited for the doctor to come in, and the first words out of his mouth were, "I have good news!" Hallelujah, I don't think I have heard those words in a long time. The doctor loaded my CT scans for the day before and the first one I had in August. The masses in August were bright white and solid spots. After four rounds of chemo, the masses are more of a gray, fluffy color and look to be breaking up. The doctor says that when they look like this, it usually means they are DEAD CELLS!!!! He couldn't say for sure because he was waiting for a blood test called a CEA to come back. This test checks how many cancer cells are in your body. In August, my CEA level was 25.8, and 3.9 is normal. This morning my CEA level came back from yesterday, and it is at 5.9!!!!! It has dropped twenty points in three months!!!!! I am two points away from normal, which means my body is doing exactly what it needs to do to FIGHT IT LIKE A BEAST!!!! With my CEA level dropping as much as it did it only backs up what the doctor thinks that they are dead cells.

The prayers and positive thoughts I have been receiving are working, and I am so thankful for them. I know I have said it before, but I couldn't have done this without all of your support!

I had round five of chemo yesterday and will be going another three rounds, making it a total of eight rounds. I talked my doctor into pushing my next round forward a week, so I didn't have to go the week of Thanksgiving and the week of Christmas. He thought the extra week off would be a good idea to help my body recover a bit before the next set of rounds. The plan so far is that my last round will be January 2, and then I will have four to six weeks off of chemo before I go into surgery, which will most likely be in March 2015. After that, will be six more weeks of recovery, and after that, there is no plan. That is fine by me... I think my head would explode going that far into next year, day by day!

If you have checked out my GoFundMe campaign recently, you will notice that after a very generous donation, I have surpassed my goal! I am truly honored and appreciative of all the support: monetary, emotional, and through prayer! The t-shirts are in, and I will be picking them up tomorrow. I will try to get them out to everyone within the next week. Thank you to all those who ordered them, and if you would still like one, I will have extras. I would love to see you all in them so if you want to post a picture of you in your "Fight Like A Beast" shirt on here or my Facebook page, that would be awesome!

I hope you are all staying warm during this very cold stretch of winter-like weather. I myself will be staying indoors as much as I can over the next few days! Too cold for this girl! Prayers and love are with you all!

All my Love,
Christine

happy thanksgiving!!!

DEC. 1, 2014, 7:42 PM

I can't believe it is already December and only twenty-four days away from Christmas. I hope everyone had a fabulous Thanksgiving and is enjoying the start of the holiday season.

Thanksgiving has always been one of my favorite holidays, but I have to admit it has always been because of the food: the pumpkin pie, the stuffing, and not to mention the turkey! But this year it means so much more to me. I am so thankful for all the family and friends that are in my life. I am thankful to God for putting all these amazing people in my life and helping me through this journey. And it feels weird to say, but I am thankful that this journey has brought me closer to my family and friends. God is truly all-powerful and has been answering our prayers. I feel amazing, and I am looking forward to my final round (as of now) of chemo on December 31st.

Last time at the doctor, I was given amazing news about my blood test and CT scan results, and the good news keeps coming. A few weeks ago (before I hit the goal on my GoFundMe site), I had applied for financial assistance from Mayo Clinic. Hoping for a payment plan, I sent in all the paperwork to avoid being sent to collections on my nearly

$2,500 bill. This morning on my way out the door, I noticed a letter, not a bill, from Mayo Clinic. I opened the letter and read that they not only accepted my application, but they also wrote off my ENTIRE bill. I do not owe a dime!!! So, the funds that have been raised will now go toward the hospital bills that will accrue in 2015 (which is already next month)! I am so thankful for everyone's support, and love that I have received and the donations toward my campaign, those who have purchased shirts, and those who ordered from my fundraiser through 31 Gifts (https://mythirtyone.com/mkarshbaum), which is still going on until December 4th if you would still like to order. :) Thank you all from the bottom of my heart and know that I thank God that you are all in my life.

All my Love,
   Christine

happy holidays!

DEC. 19, 2014, 11:50 AM

Wow! I can't believe how fast this month is going. I am currently on round seven of eight, with my last round going to be on New Year's Eve. Round six was a little rough, and I ended up getting sick at home, so the doctor did some switching of the medications I receive, and it helped this round. I still got a little nauseous, but it wasn't as bad or did not last as long, thank goodness. Erbert's and Gerbert's delivers until 3:00 am, cause around 10:00 pm I was starving! Once my final round is done, I will be going in for a surgery consult in the second week of January and planning on surgery being in March. I have to be off of chemo for two months before I can go through surgery. I have been keeping really busy and have had lots of energy, seeing as my iron level is up to 11.9 (12.1 is normal). I have made all sorts of goodies and put up the tree. I am planning on decorating the tree, icing the sugar cookies and gingerbread men, and wrapping the gifts for under the tree. I don't know if I will get it all done today, but definitely by Sunday. I have a few sewing projects left to do for gifts, but otherwise, I am pretty much done with my Christmas shopping.

Earlier this week I had made one of my chemo nurses a pair of mustache scrubs, and I brought all the staff a tin full of cookies. Before I was even done with chemo at the clinic, they had finished the whole tin! I also included a card to let them know how thankful I am for the work they do. Seeing as we have a few nurses in the family, I know that they don't always get the recognition they deserve, and I wanted to make sure they heard it from me.

This is the time of year to remember what is important in life. Giving is truly better than receiving, but it doesn't have to be giving of gifts; it can be giving your time as well. I plan on volunteering at the food bank this Christmas and bringing those who are less fortunate some happiness and joy. When the holiday season first started, I didn't feel like decorating the house or putting up the tree, and then I thought, "If this were my last Christmas, would I do it differently?" Now, I do not under any circumstances believe this is my last Christmas, but the answer was Yes. So, I got the tree up and opened up the Christmas decorations box. Between baking and decorating, I instantly felt my mood get better, and the Christmas spirit was upon me. It's easy to get caught up in all the hoopla of this time of year, but please remember the reason for the season!

All my Love,
Christine

final round of my battle royale

DEC. 31, 2014, 1:59 AM

Here it is, the night before what will hopefully be my last round of chemo. As you can see, sleep is not coming as easily tonight, although it usually doesn't the night before a treatment. It's hard to believe the holidays are almost at an end, and a new year will be starting soon. I was fortunate to be able to spend my Christmas with family and was able to enjoy my mini-vacation from work. I have another five days off starting tomorrow, which is great because starting next week, I am full-time again at work for the next two months. I am looking forward to going back to a normal schedule again. I will still be a floater at work, but it will be nice to be able to work Monday through Friday again. Boy, I never thought I would say that before all this started.

Thank you for all the well-wishes and beautiful Christmas cards I have received. I hope everyone had a wonderful Christmas and had their fill of Christmas goodies. I know I did. Don't worry, Aunt Julie, I will drop off your peanut butter balls at Grandma's before I go to chemo.;) I made way too many cookies this year, but was happy to be able to give them to friends and family. Dad even needed a second batch... I told him to go for the big tin the first time. Haha.

I have been thinking a lot about my New Year's resolution, as I can't really use my old standby of losing weight. I have put on about twenty pounds since starting chemo, but I will need that buffer for when I go into surgery, as the last time I was in the hospital for a week; that's about how much I lost by the time I was discharged. So, this coming year, I will be focusing on two things. The first is eating clean, as my attempts have fallen by the wayside since being able to eat dairy again (I'm pretty sure the twenty-pound weight gain is all from cheese, haha). With the last round of chemo being tomorrow, I want to focus on detoxing my body and making it stronger. Surgery can do a number on your body, and I want to be as healthy as I can be before going into that operating room. If anyone has any tips or advice on this, I am all ears, as I am not even 100% sure what all consists of eating clean, but I did get some books from the library. Haha.

And second, I want to focus on living for others. God obviously has a plan for me, and I guess I wasn't paying attention after the first wake-up call He gave me. Through this journey, I have been given clarity on so many choices in my life and have been able to know what I want from life as I am now fighting for it. It's kind of like how people say if you need to make a choice, flip a coin, and when the coin is in the air, you will know which way you are leaning. I know what I am missing in life, and I know what is important now. I have always believed in God and considered myself a Christian, but it wasn't until recently that I under-stood what being a Christian entailed. Apparently, the twelve years I spent in Catholic school never made it click. To me, being a Christian is loving your neighbor, caring for your neighbor, and clothing your neighbor. Jesus said that when we do this for our neighbors, we are doing this for Him. I wasn't able to volunteer on Christmas Day at the community table because I wasn't feeling well, but it is something I want to start doing. If anyone wants to come with me... let me know! And also I am going to be volunteering some of my time at the Wellness Shack, where my dad works. I'm not sure how much help I can be to the people who come in, but I hear my organizational skills could come in handy;)

Well, that's all for tonight. I will update you all this weekend on what Dr. C has planned for the next two months and what my CEA level comes back as. Stay warm as Mother Nature throws her hissy fit for the next week or so. I will be staying indoors as much as I can for the next five days.

All my Love,
Christine

2015

5....4....3....2....1 happy new year!

JAN. 1, 2015, 1:52 PM

Round eight is officially in progress, and it started out a little rough. I went into it nauseated, and it only got worse. I didn't throw up, but I was nauseous until around eleven. The fact that it was my last round is what got me through it. By this morning, I was eating toast and eggs and even had a sub for lunch. Yesterday, when I met with my doctor, he told me my iron is up to 12.9, and we found out my CEA level is down to 3.6; anything under four is normal.

So, the next step is my surgery consult on January 13. This appointment will decide whether the next step is surgery or radiation. If surgery is the next step, I could be going as soon as the end of January, not the beginning of March. Which means I could be back at work by the middle to end of March.

I received a lot of gifts from my nurses yesterday as well as a bottle of sparkling cider and a certificate for completing my last round of chemo. I will miss seeing them every other week, but I will be back for doctor's visits every now and then.

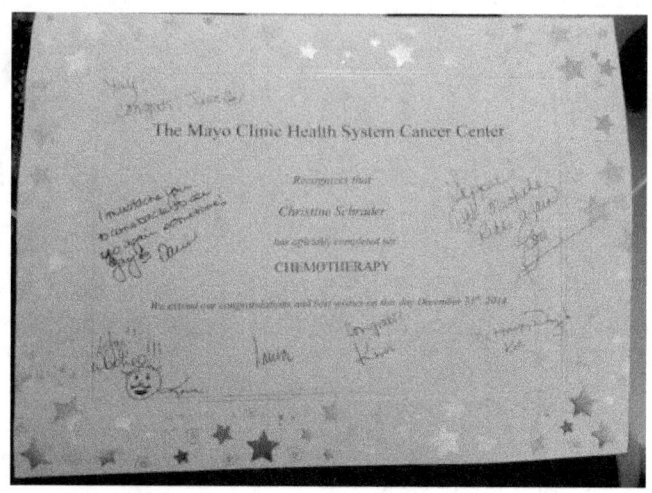

I hope everyone had a great New Year's Eve and is enjoying the first day of 2015. I'm glad it's not below zero here, but I still have no intention of leaving the house until tomorrow to get my pump off. I can't believe it's already my last round and that my body has responded so well to the treatments. To go from a CEA level of 25 to 3 only four months later is amazing, and I give it all up to God. I know I would not have done so well without your prayers and support.

All my Love,
　Christine

"when you die, it does not mean that you lose to cancer. you beat cancer by how you live, why you live, and in the manner in which you live." -stuart scott

JAN. 13, 2015, 5:10 PM

Wow! Has time flown by or what?!? The holidays have come and gone, and once again all we are left with is... SNOW and COLD! Last week was pretty brutal for the weather here in WI, but I am happy to announce that my cold sensitivity is gone and the last round of chemo has left my body! I still have most of my hair (which now that chemo is out of my body will hopefully start growing back in), my positive attitude, an amazing energy level, and the love and support from hundreds of friends and family!

Today I went to my surgery consult, as this was the next step in my treatment plan. I received news that I didn't want to hear but was prepared for. The general surgeon (the same one that was a ray of sunshine the first time I met him and told me "good luck" before HE operated on me) told me that he was having a hard time deciding whether he would do the surgery because it was so controversial.

Controversial in the fact that even if he did the surgery that he was not curing me, and that I still had cancer. There's the sunshine again... just beaming. Oh, it gets better! Then he told me that the cancer in my lungs and liver would be what killed me before the colorectal cancer did. Now, to talk about what surgery he would be performing. After a very uncomfortable exam (yep, think about the location of my cancer. I will never complain about my yearly "ladies" doctor appointment ever again!), he informed me that although the masses have shrunk and are softer that the only way to remove the affected area would to take out the entire section and leave me with a colostomy bag. So, I did what any rational twenty-nine-year-old woman would do facing swimsuit season... I asked for a referral for a second opinion from a colorectal surgeon down in Rochester! There is no way I am not getting a second and possibly even a third opinion on a surgery that will impact my life for the rest of my life! Sooooooo, surgery is currently postponed until I can find someone to tell me what I want to hear. Haha. I'm stubborn like that; just ask my dad! I haven't set up the referral appointment, but when I do, I will let you all know.

A few weeks ago, a friend passed along the link to a YouTube video about a "Cancer-Fighting Salad." I took a look at it then and kind of put it out of my mind. With everything else going on, I wasn't prepared to overhaul my diet, as well as the fact that I was extremely nervous to change anything while on chemo in case it stopped working. But with my New Year's resolution to start eating clean, I decided to go back and check it out again. I hate eating the same thing over and over, but if it will help my chances to beat this, I will suck it and DO IT! I mean the salad even has zucchini on it, and I HATE zucchini. Just ask my mom! While watching the video, I saw that this guy had a website, chrisbeat-cancer.com. Now, if that isn't a sign from God, I don't know what is. What made my jaw drop to the floor is that Chris was diagnosed with stage 3 colorectal cancer at age twenty-six! His site is very inspirational and informative. I encourage you all to watch his video, which is on the main page. He talks about his journey and why he chose to change his lifestyle in order to survive. I have started this week to eat clean, and I have already learned so much from what I have read. The benefits of eating unprocessed food are astronomical, and I can't wait to be on a completely clean diet. It feels so much different this time as opposed to the other times I have tried to diet for weight loss. I am not concerned with counting calories or depriving myself of that piece of chocolate. This is strictly for health reasons, and it makes it a little easier to follow it that way. I don't want anyone to feel like I am pushing my "Uber healthy diet" on you. I am concerned only for my family and friends. The last thing I want is to have anyone else go through the battle that I am going through.

And finally. Last week, we lost a great man, Stuart Scott. He was an announcer on SportsCenter and a cancer survivor. Mr. Scott was diagnosed with cancer in 2004 and beat it. He beat it again in 2007 when it reared its nasty head, and again he went to battle when it showed up in 2014. This man is an inspiration and a huge motivation in my life. He talks about how after he had a chemo treatment of 5FU (the same drug I was on), he would feel extreme queasiness. I could have put it better myself, but he didn't retreat to the bed or couch; he would go and do a P90X routine. If you do not know what P90X is, it is an intense workout that lasts usually 60-90 minutes... I couldn't even do it when I was healthy! We are talking right after chemo... not an hour or two or even a day, but right after! He felt that every time he would work out, even though he felt like garbage, he was telling cancer "FU" (Sorry Grandma, his words, not mine :)). I could barely even get off the couch, and this man was at the gym... chemo pump in tow! Wow! I felt so inspired when I read his story, but it was what he said at an award ceremony after receiving a perseverance award that really stuck with me. He said, "When you die, it does not mean that you lose to cancer. You beat cancer by how you live, why you live, and in the manner in which you live." I mean, WOW! What strength and determination he had. And this is why I do what I do. This is why I still work as close to full-time as I can, why I have a positive attitude, why I "Fight It Like A Beast!" Cause Mr. Scott was a beast and he fought for his life!!!

All my Love,
Christine

life doesn't have a remote... you need to get up to change it

JAN. 29, 2015, 10:56 PM

Tonight is the night before my second opinion in Rochester. Sue Ann drove up this afternoon, and together we drove down to Rochester after I was done with work. I have two appointments tomorrow, and will keep everyone posted on the outcomes of those. It's strange, but I am oddly calm, where the night before the last consult, I was a ball of nerves. Hopefully, that is a good omen. Lots of prayer helps, too.

All my Love,
Christine

warning! the following update is extremely honest and may contain issues that are uncomfortable!

JAN. 31, 2015, 5:53 PM

Yesterday was my second opinion in Rochester. My first appointment was with the physician's assistant to go over my case and to have a physical. She would then present her findings to the colorectal surgeon and go from there. My second appointment was with the colorectal surgeon. After talking to her physician's assistant, she presented her findings to me. I have to say that both of them really impressed me with their demeanor and the understanding that they showed me. It only took a few minutes for me to know that they are truly looking out for my well-being. During my consult with the surgeon, she went over the findings of my exam (same as Dr. Erickson's). She made sure that I understood each and every finding and answered every question I had. Unfortunately, her findings were that the only way to do the surgery is to end in a colostomy bag. Even if the masses dissolve with radiation, the chance of it coming back is extremely high. So, her opinion is that we start radiation and then do surgery so that the chance of recurrence is lower. This alone was a lot to take in, but there's more.

Starting radiation would consist of having it Monday through

Friday for fifteen minutes each day... every day for six weeks. During this time, I would be receiving 5FU (the chemo drug) as well. There would be a six-week break after radiation before surgery would start. During this six-week break, I would be put back on my full-dose of chemo, which is 5FU, as well as the two other chemo drugs. This was too much to take in at one time, and I began to break down. I couldn't stop crying, and I just wanted to get out of there as fast as I could. The surgeon wants me to see a medical oncologist and a radiation oncologist as well to go over the best way to do the radiation and chemo. There is talk of doing a shorter version of radiation, where it would only be five days of radiation (one full week), and then surgery would happen the next week. The radiation would be more intense, and there is a greater chance of recurrence. So, I will be heading back down to Rochester in two weeks (Feb. 9). They want to start this process very soon, so I will have more doctor's appointments in the next few weeks.

After all my information was updated, and appointments were scheduled, SueAnn and I headed home. The whole way home, I went through a lot of emotions; fear, anger, depression, etc. Silent tears streamed down my face as I drove and there was little talking. When we would talk about the opinion we had just received, I would go into a panic and become agitated and start to get the sweats. At one point I just started yelling, "I can't talk about this. Non-stop talking, I can't do this right now." My sister is a saint, for all that we went through that day! We met Sarah at I.C. (Immaculate Conception, my old elementary school and parish) for the fish boil. Let me tell you, Sarah is the queen of distraction. By the time we had sat down to eat, I was feeling better.

We decided to go to a movie, but had some time to kill before it started, so we went to have some adult beverages... something we all agreed we had earned that day. They knew I didn't want to talk about what had gone on that day, and so the conversations were a bit forced. Once again, I began to go over the information I had received that day, and the emotional roller coaster began again. At one point in time, I had to go to the bathroom because I could feel the tears starting. The rest of the night was better, and any tears I had were from laughing too hard... *The Wedding Singer* is hilarious! Well... it was better until I got home. I don't know what it is about being home, but I became completely unglued. I started sobbing uncontrollably, and it lasted a good twenty minutes. I knew sleep wasn't going to be an option with all the thoughts going through my head, especially the one that caused the most damage, "I can't do this!" Chemo was hard enough the first eight rounds; how was I going to be able to do another three to four, knowing exactly how it was going to be with the nausea, cold sensitivity, and other symptoms. Funny movies are the best distractions for me (except for Sarah;)) so we put in a movie and I eventually fell asleep due to sleep exhaustion.

The next morning, I woke up and my eyes resembled goldfish lips. Haha. But I felt a lot better. I didn't feel as defeated as I had the day before. And then I was reading my Facebook feed, and a story of a little girl who went to my Child Care OH Center came up. She had been diagnosed the month before I had with leukemia and was currently in treatment. As I read her story and the updates her mom had been adding, I started thinking. This is a three-year-old who has been through so much in the last six months. She was on a much more aggressive type of chemo and was now rocking a shaved head. She was affected a lot more by her treatments with vomiting, pain, etc., and all through this, every single picture I found of her, she had a smile on! Little Miss Ellis, you are an inspiration! I had been trying to find inspiration in books, stories, etc., and all I had to do was look in the face of this sweet, loving child. It was at that very moment that my "I can't do this" changed to "I GOT THIS!"

Thank you for all the prayers and positive thoughts being sent my way. I do apologize for the delay on the update, but it took a few days to process before I was able to journal exactly what I was thinking and feeling. I hope everyone is doing well and that you all have a great week!

All my Love,
Christine

some days you're the pigeon, some days you're the statue

FEB. 9, 2015, 7:00 AM

It was brought to my attention that I had put the wrong date for my next doctor's appointment. It is not today, but next Monday, the sixteenth. I will keep you all posted on what happens. On a short note, please keep my family in your prayers. My 107-year-old great-grandma passed away Friday night. I had only met her a handful of times, but she sure was an amazing lady. My dad was saying how it was going to be a small funeral because she had outlived all her friends, but then I reminded him of our large family. She had forty grandchildren, ninety-eight great-grandchildren, and forty-eight great-great-grandchildren. It's gonna be a packed house.

Have a great week and remember what you're grateful for!

All my Love,
Christine

carpe diem

FEB. 23, 2015, 9:40 PM

Many apologies for being so extremely late with this journal update. I have been working a lot and enjoyed doing nothing this last weekend!

Last Monday, I had two doctor's appointments down in Rochester. The first was with a radiology oncologist, and the other was with a medical oncologist. The first appointment was to go over the two different courses of radiation before surgery. The short course, which would be five days in a row with surgery to follow the next week, or the long course, which would be five days a week for five and a half weeks. After talking to the doctor, I was swaying more toward the short course. There are fewer side effects and less nerve damage done. Regardless of the course I choose, it will fry my ovaries and, chances are, put me into pre-menopause. Now, I have to think about freezing my eggs and talking to a fertility specialist. By the end of this appointment, my head was spinning. I pretty much stopped listening. It seems like every doctor's appointment I go to, the opinion changes. At this point, my mind is spinning, and I am starting to come to the realization that this surgery could happen in the next month.

The time until the next appointment lasted forever. I first met with the oncologist's nurse practitioner, and she went over my diagnosis and treatment plan thus far. She asked me whether I had had certain tests, and she asked me about why certain decisions were made for treatment. She gave me a quick physical and told me that my kidneys and liver felt really good and healthy. She stepped out, and the oncologist came in, Dr. Grothey (pronounced *growthy*) horrible name for an oncologist. Dr. Grothey asked me more questions about the care I had been receiving and why I hadn't had a scan in over three months, even after I had requested one. He looked at me and asked, "Why are you going through with this surgery?"

Ummmm... what? Come again? I informed him that I had been under the understanding that I had to get it done. He informed me that my odds didn't get better with the surgery or worse without it. I was going to put myself through a life-altering surgery for nothing except a huge risk of complications during it. My jaw hit the floor. I was completely speechless.

"I am very concerned with the care you have been receiving in Eau Claire." He told me. There is a great chemo drug that works extremely well with the drugs I was already on. This new drug searches for cells that have too many blood vessels attached to them (a key trait of cancer cells) and kills these blood vessels. Basically, making it a cancer-killing machine. He was very confused about why I was taken off treatment when I was reacting so well to it, and he was dumbfounded that a scan had not been done since November even though I had requested one at the end of December. "I don't get my way a lot... just ask my wife. But I want you to transfer your care down the Rochester so I am able to oversee it."

Dr. Grothey told me that he has seen many patients my age with colorectal cancer, including a fifteen-year-old! So it was the easiest choice I have made since this whole process started. I had prayed for guidance and clarity just that morning on the way down to Rochester, and I really felt that this was where I needed to be. No surgery? Is this possible? No colostomy bag? Another summer in a two-piece? PRAISE JESUS!!!!

I transferred my care to Rochester, and I was immediately scheduled the next day for blood work, and CT scan, and another consult with Dr.

Grothey's nurse practitioner, Jessica. Sarah and Sue Ann both had to work on Tuesday, so we all drove back, and I would drive up the next day to go to these appointments. Dan heard that I was going alone, and he called in to work in order to take me. The next morning, we had to leave at 6:00 am, and I slept the whole way up. I hadn't been getting a lot of sleep at this time due to anxiety about my doctor's appointments, so any sleep I could get, I was taking. After the blood work was done, I had my CT scan. In Eau Claire, this is a very... uncomfortable task. So have to drink thirty-two ounces of a very disgusting drink (second only to the taste of a colonoscopy prep) in forty-five minutes and then you are taking to an absolutely freezing room where you are passed through a doughnut-shaped machine multiple times while holding your breath throughout the fifteen to twenty-minute scan while a dye is injected into your vein that makes you feel like you have wet your pants! In Rochester, however, you drink sixteen ounces of PLAIN water in ten minutes and are passed through the doughnut-shaped machine once. Five minutes and I was done!!!

During my consult, I went over a lot of stuff with Jessica (my new favorite person at Rochester), and in one afternoon (three hours actually), she had gone through both scans and compared them, so I was able to see the differences between the scan in November and Tuesday's scan. Meeting her and Dr. Grothey has given me the confidence in my treatment and in the fact that I am on the right path. The scans showed that the masses in my lungs have started to grow back and that one of the two masses on my liver is slightly bigger. The other liver mass is considerably smaller, and the rectal masses have shrunk drastically. So it was a good news/bad news scenario, but I was really glad to know exactly what was going on in my body. I asked her whether I had any limitations, as I really want to start running again.

She looked at me like I was crazy and, with a smile, said, "Go For It!" There was a study that looked at those with rectal cancer who were stationary vs. those who walked sixty minutes a day six days a week, and those who walked had slower-growing masses than those who didn't. I am also off my iron pills and on a multivitamin. When I asked her about teas, herbs, and other natural "cancer fighters" I had been told about, she told me that the best thing I can do for my body right now is to eat well, exercise, and take a multivitamin. So, I am going to continue to eat clean, and once my gym opens next week, I will be working out five times a week. The current plan for my treatment is to start back on chemo on Thursday and to add the new drug. They are also going to teach Dan and me how to take off the pump so I am able to do this at home, versus going to urgent care to get it taken off. They are just so handy in Rochester. They are revamping my anti-nausea medications to help with that side effect, as I told them it was really the only side effect I really hate.

Welcome to the roller coaster of emotions I have been going through over the last week. I think it took a good three days for it to sink in that I wasn't going to have surgery, and even now, I have trouble believing it. Once the weather is warm, I am planning a trip to Noah's Ark as well as a trip to Las Vegas this summer for my 30th BIRTHDAY! Before all this started, I was dreading turning thirty, and now I am blessed that I am alive for another birthday. We don't know when our number is up; it could be tomorrow, next week, a year from now, ten years, fifty... no one knows. Tell the ones you love how much they mean to you, do something that scares you, and take chances. Live today for you and those around you... BE PRESENT! None of these sayings made any sense until now, and I am glad I understand them now. I know what's important to me, and I know I want to enjoy my life.

All my Love,
Christine

no one fights alone!

The next part of this journey started yesterday with my ninth round of chemo. Yesterday started with an appointment with a geneticist to go over my family history and to start the process of genetic testing in order to understand more of how I got here and what information they can find in order to properly screen family members. She sent me down for a blood test, and I will get the results in the next three to four weeks. I will also be meeting with a geneticist around this same time to discuss the genetic testing for my long QT syndrome.

Once I was done with this appointment, I realized how nervous I was for the chemo appointment I had later in the afternoon. Of the symptoms that I have with chemo, it is the nausea that really does me in. It only lasts a few hours, but it is so intense that it is a hindrance to my wanting to get treatment. With this round, it was going to be some new drugs as well as a new routine. Instead of getting three anti-nausea medications, I will only be getting two and will no longer be getting Lorazepam and Reglan. Lorazepam makes me feel all drugged up and causes me to sleep during the entire session. With all these changes, I was most worried that my nausea was going to either be the same or worse. Dan met me at the hospital before my chemo started, and we got lunch. I had always been opposed to eating before chemo, after I threw up the first round, but I thought it might help if I had food in my stomach. I made myself eat a sandwich about an hour before chemo and hoped that it would make a difference. Within no time, it was time for chemo, and I walked through the doors with a ball of nerves in my stomach. The nurses are all really nice, and two of them were actually UWEC graduates. My nausea always started an hour before chemo ended, so it was a waiting game to see what would happen. The time finally came. I had an hour left on my chemo drugs... it was go time! I had been snacking on some saltines and drinking tea, and as the time ticked away, I did not have any nausea at all! Not even a twinge of it, and I didn't feel drugged up at all. It was the first time I had ever walked out of a treatment and not felt in a fog. I was feeling so good that I could have gone for some Chinese food! But I didn't. I can't even imagine what that would have done to my body after eating clean for so many weeks. So I still get the pump to wear for the next two days, but this time it is an automated pump, quite a bit larger than the one I had before. Let's put it this way: when I put on my sweatshirt to go get breakfast at the hotel this morning, I looked about six months pregnant. I got quite a few looks walking through the hotel lobby this morning. I named my "chemo baby" Larry (if you have seen the show "Impractical Jokers," you know who I named it after. Haha), and they showed Dan and me how to take it off, so no more driving an hour for a five-minute appointment at urgent care to get it off. So now I am back home with no nausea and no fatigue, and just able to enjoy the day. Because I am going back to work full time in a room, I have moved my treatments to Fridays and will be putting myself on bed rest on the weekends I have treatment. This is just an added way to make sure I am fully rested to make it through the next week with our thirteen three-year-olds! I am definitely open to a few visitors during these weekends... hint, hint!

So this round I did it a little differently than I usually do. Instead of a mustache, I wore bracelets, one for each type of cancer that I am battling or that I know someone who has it or battled it. White for lung cancer, which I lost both of my grandpas to, Teal/Pink/Purple for thyroid cancer for a friend who is now cancer-free, blue for yours truly, orange for leukemia for a special little girl named Ellis and my friend Katie Lee who we lost almost ten years ago, and pink for breast cancer for a friend who is now cancer-free. The bands say, "No one fights alone," and it is so true.

Not only do I have so many people who are fighting the battle themselves, but I have so many friends and family who have brought themselves into my battle with their support and love. And not to mention that I have God on my side. He has been beside me since the beginning, and I know that he will never leave my side. And to show my support for a special little girl during her fight, I will be going to the Ellis Paulson Benefit on Sunday, March 1st, from 1:00 pm to 6:00 pm at the Eagles Club in Hallie. I would encourage anyone and everyone to join me for a great cause. If you want more info, please click on the link https:// www.facebook.com/EllisPaulson There will be food (two adult meals with each raffle ticket), lots of raffle prizes, games for the kids, and so much more! Hope to see you there!

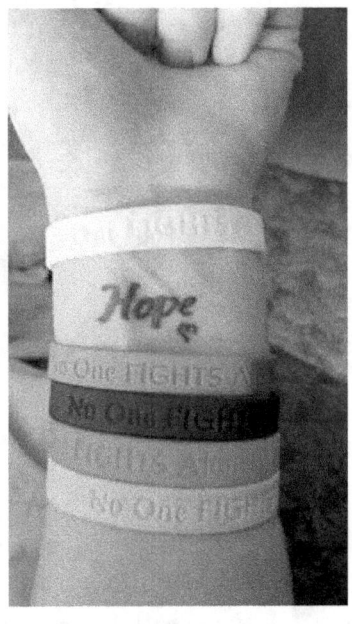

All my Love,
Christine

"she is clothed in strength and dignity and laughs with no fear of the future." -proverbs 31:25

MAR. 14, 2015, 7:33 AM

Well, it's official! The funk that has inhabited my body since January has left and been replaced by the Rockstar that started this journey!!!!

The second round of chemo is in full swing, and like the last, I have absolutely no nausea. I met with my oncologist's nurse practitioner, Jessica, yesterday prior to starting chemo, to go over my lab results. She was extremely impressed with how I did with my last round, especially because she had given me the maximum dose she could. I told her that cold sensitivity was the only side effect I really had and that the tingling in my toes lasted the whole two weeks. She had told me that it was due to my receiving the maximum dose and that she could come down on it a little to help with it. I told her, "No way! I can deal with it, and I have felt so good after the last round that we should just keep it the way it was." My lab results were all normal, including the liver test that was slightly high last round. She was so happy with the aftermath of my first round and was really happy to be able to keep going with the treatment plan we had all agreed on. I did have a low-grade fever when I went in yesterday, but I do believe I am beginning to get a sinus infection. Thursday night, I had a headache with lots of pressure behind my eyes, across my forehead, and at the base of my skull. Due to my long QT syndrome, I cannot take antihistamines, and because of the cancer, I cannot take ibuprofen because it's a blood thinner. Sarah stayed the night on Thursday because she was coming with me to my appointments the next day. She was amazing and gave me a face massage to help drain some of the pressure I was having. It did help a little, but I was still having the headache yesterday when I went in to see the doctor. I am sure sleep deprivation and dehydration were partly the issue as well. She was hesitant to give me antibiotics, but said she could, seeing as I can't take anything over the counter. Seeing as the headache only started the night before, I did not feel antibiotics were necessary.

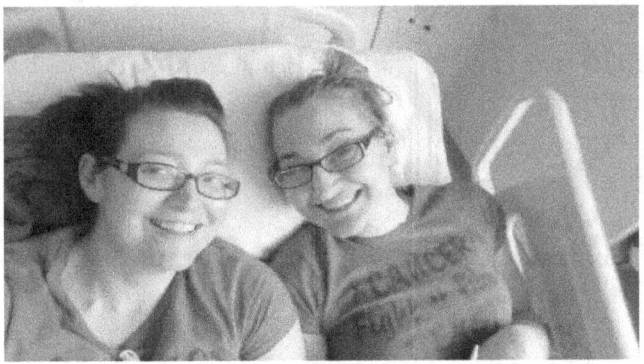

Sarah gave me another massage after we got home, and the pressure is a lot less than it was yesterday. A few rounds with a hot pack should kick this out of my system. For my chemo appointment, because Dan and Sarah were with me, they gave us a private room with a bed. Sarah was sleep-deprived as well, so I let her get in the bed with me. It took them a while to get my drugs set up, so we were about an hour behind. The chemo itself only took two and a half hours, which is a huge improvement from the rounds I did in Eau Claire. As the nurse was getting me set up, she asked if Sarah and I were sisters or friends. When I responded that we were sisters, she got a smile on her face and replied, "I'm glad that my girls will eventually like each other." Haha. Ain't that the truth! Sarah and I used to fight all the time, and then five minutes later, be curled up on the couch together. This drove my dad crazy when we were growing up. We had bought some cheese and caramel popcorn before chemo, and I was so hungry that I started nibbling on it during chemo (which is a first), and as chemo went on, I started eating more and more of it. This was either going to be a good idea or a really bad one! Turns out it was a good idea. I got through the entire treatment without any nausea or vomiting! SUCCESS!! Finally! And just to test this out, my GPS decided to take us on the curviest and hilliest way home. Dan was actually feeling queasy, and I was fine, not a touch of nausea! I was able to eat fine once we got home, and even though I slept an hour or two during chemo, I fell asleep at 10:00 pm and slept until 6:00 this morning. I woke with the occasional toss and turn due to the fact that I was on the couch, and I can't sleep on my belly because of the chemo pump (I'm a belly sleeper through and through). But I am still sticking with the bed rest for the weekend, and, fingers crossed, will be back to full energy by Monday morning. Those three-year-olds don't stop for anything!

Just a heads up, but I will be starting a group for The Color Run on May 17th in Carson Park. I ran it last year, only three months before being diagnosed, and I feel way better than I did then. I will give you all more info about it after I get it all set up. I hope you are all enjoying this warm weather and taking advantage of it.

All my Love,
Christine

happy easter

APR. 7, 2015, 8:40 PM

I can't believe that is has been three weeks since I had a journal entry. I guess it's a good thing that nothing has really happened. Haha. On March 27th, I had my eleventh round of chemo (third in Rochester), and everything went great. There was no nausea, fatigue, and barely any cold sensitivity. I was able to eat during treatment and had lunch right after. This is still such a huge accomplishment over what I was experiencing before.

Saturday after treatment, I was on bed rest, but Sunday I was going all day. The child care center I work at was having a bake/craft sale the next week, and there were some things I wanted to do for it. The center had decided that they wanted the proceeds from the bake/craft sale to go to me to help with travel expenses back and forth from Rochester. I could not believe it; I felt so loved and supported. Just when I thought I couldn't feel more loved the two-day sale came to a close with a whopping $844 raised!!!!! My jaw hit the floor, and I could not believe how lucky I was to be working in such an amazing place where I had so much support behind me from the staff and families. I do feel like everyone there is a part of my family, and I couldn't imagine working in a better place than I do right now. On a side note... if you are reading this and you were a part of this amazing gift, please let me say thank you from the bottom of my heart. I truly believe that I am going to get the best possible care in Rochester, and it is comforting to know that I do not have to worry about my expenses to get to and from my doctors.

Last weekend I went to Chicago to see my sister and her family for Easter. It was great to have a couple of days with the family and to be able to dye eggs and have an egg hunt with the girls. However, now I feel a little behind on what I wanted to get done this week. I started back at the gym this week and have gone twice so far. I plan to go five days this week, as well as before treatment on Friday. I have signed up for The Color Run next month and have a long way to go before I am ready to run that 5K. I have set up a group for the run and invite anyone who wants to have the time of their life to join! The group is called "Fight Like A Beast," and the run is on May 17th. Let me know if you have any questions.

I hope everyone is well and that we will all be enjoying some spring weather soon! 🩶

All my Love,
Christine

silver lining

APR. 20, 2015, 8:13 PM

It's hard to believe that this entire journey started eight months ago today! Sometimes it feels like it's been well over a year, and on other days it feels like I just found out. Well, let me catch you up on what has happened this month. On April 10th, I had my twelfth round of chemo, and it started without any issues. While getting my blood drawn for my labs, the nurse was asking me what round I was on. When I replied twelfth, she got a concerned look on her face. She informed me that after the tenth round; they watch for allergic reactions to one of the chemo drugs I take and let me know the symptoms. Well, what do ya know... guess who had an allergic reaction? Yep, ME!!! I started to have itching on my palms, and my whole body went flush. They immediately stopped my treatment (I was almost done anyway) and gave me some Benadryl. Once the itching stopped, they restarted the other chemo drug and let me finish it. I just have to keep things interesting! Haha. The rest of the round went well. I had little fatigue and no nausea, with a fairly good appetite. So now that my fourth round in Rochester was done, the next step was a CT scan and a meeting with the doctor. The scheduling progress proved to be a bit of a hassle this time around as I was unable to get all my appointments done on the same day. Originally, I was to have four appointments in Rochester over three days. Knowing that I could not afford to miss that much work, I called and called until they were able to get everything scheduled in two days instead of three—still not the best, but definitely better.

So this morning was my CT scan and consult with my doctor. Because the scans take a bit, I had labs and the scan in the morning, and my consult was in the afternoon. After Sarah and I got some lunch, we were both tired, as we were up at the gym by 6:30 this morning, so we decided to take a snooze in the car before we went in for the CAT scan consult. It was pretty bright out, so we put on jackets and sweatshirts to make a car fort. Haha. A fifteen-minute nap is all I got, and soon it was time to go see the doctor. I had not seen Dr. Jessica in over a month, and I was eager to know the results of the scan. She came in with a huge smile and said, "They look great!" We went over the scans, and she showed me that the two spots on my liver have gotten smaller and that she couldn't even see anything on my lymph nodes. After looking at the spots on my lungs, you could see that a lot of them had shrunk and that a good number of them had started to have black spots in the middle, so they looked like doughnuts. Dr. Jessica informed me that this means they are dying from the inside out! A sign. We then talked about the fact that I had an allergic reaction to the chemo drug, and she said that I could no longer take that drug, and we would have to switch it out with a new one. Now this is good and suck-y news (I didn't want to use "bad" cause it's more of just a setback), because the drug that I can no longer take is the drug that gives me the cold sensitivity (hello ice cream and popsicles this summer), but the one that they are switching me to will most likely thin out my hair so much that I will lose all my hair. Which definitely sucks, but knowing that my body is doing so well in fighting this, I guess I will give up some hair for the chance to "Fight It Like A Beast!"

Silver lining... I don't have to shave my legs this summer! :) It's not the best outcome, but like everything else, I will prepare myself for what will happen next and move on. A poor attitude will not change anything, but a positive attitude will make life more fun! Plus, now Ellis and I will have even more in common as we had "Show and Tell" with our ports on Friday. So I got a prescription for a wig, and I am going to make some scarves to wear. After we went over everything, Dr. Jessica asked me how I was going to cope with losing my hair (a question I could tell she asks a lot), and I looked at her and said, "Cut it short until it falls out, and then wear a scarf or wig."

A smile came across her face, and she asked me, "How are you so positive through all this?"

My response was, "I don't know." Haha. I honestly don't know how I am; it was more like a switch that flipped. All I know is, the better I feel, the better my treatment goes. We talked about it for a while, and she told me that for most of her day she is helping patients cope with their diagnoses and get through depression. She said that she is going to tell her other patients about me and my story. I felt so honored that she wanted to tell my story to be able to help others who are in the same boat as me.

So that was my Monday. After running a mile and a half, driving for over four hours and over four hours of doctor's appointments, I am exhausted and am heading to bed.

Just a reminder that The Color Run is on May 17th and if you would like to join our team, it's called Fight Like A Beast.

All my Love,
Christine

round 13... good thing i'm not superstitious

APR. 27, 2015

Well, the thirteenth round has been completed, and all my worries were put to rest as I had no new side effects. Sarah and I headed down to Rochester on Friday afternoon and were all set to start the new drug that was switched out due to my allergic reaction last round. There was some talk previously about doing an anti-sensitizing process, but that would mean I would have to be hospitalized, and my two and a half to three-hour treatment would be more like an eight-hour treatment. I was up for it, but my doctor didn't want to put me through it, seeing as it wasn't a sure thing that it would work. So, she wanted to start me on a new drug that will most likely continue to thin my hair until it's gone, not the greatest outcome, but I am down for it if it will continue to destroy the cancer in my body. Some of this is a recap from the last update, so just bear with me. Needless to say, I was extremely nervous heading into this round, as I wasn't sure how well my body was going to react to the new regimen. I had done so well in the first twelve rounds. Yeah, I had some tough days, but nothing like I have heard about with other patients. I was nauseous in the beginning, but only for part of a day. What if, with this new drug, I am sick all the time or so tired I couldn't go to work? Let me tell you something... the "What If?" game will drive you crazy!

So, I did what I always do... I prayed. I prayed that God gave me the strength to tolerate this round just as well as the last and that he was with me to give me peace... I was just getting used to eating before, during, and after treatment. So, I followed the same regimen that I had before treatment. I would eat one to two hours prior to treatment, and then I would eat crackers slowly throughout the treatment. I got a treat this round, as it was the chemo drug they switched out that gave me cold sensitivity. Yep, that means this girl got to sip ginger ale during treatment... COLD ginger ale! It's the little things in life! :) With uncertainty about how this round would go, I booked a hotel for the night as my new drug, Irinotecan, has a nickname by other patients called "Run-to-the-can." Yeah, not the best side effect for a ninety-minute drive through the country.

On a side note, I find it very humorous how open I am with this, as I was not like this prior to eight months ago. I guess telling doctor after doctor and nurse after nurse will make it seem like not such a big deal.

Anyway, back to treatment. Once I started, they warned me of some side effects that most people had, and that if I started to have them, they could give a drug to reverse the effects, and would give me this drug before each treatment as a precaution. And what do you know? I started to have the symptoms—stomach cramps, runny nose, and a thickening of my saliva (which was the worst, but the COLD ginger ale helped). So I got this miracle shot, and all the symptoms went away. So now it was just a waiting game... when would these other side effects go to rear their heads? Well, I made it through treatment just like I had the previous four rounds, and nothing new presented.

We left the cancer center and headed to the car for our bags. I was feeling a bit sweaty (a known side effect), and I was STARVING! I just wanted to get into the hotel room and eat some food! If you have never been to Rochester Mayo before, it is an amazing maze of sublevels and skyways. We were able to walk from the hospital to the parking ramp and then to the hotel without ever having to step outside, which was nice because it was raining all day! I didn't know what I wanted to eat, but I knew something light but filling was in my near future. We talked a lot about what we were hungry for, and I finally decided that we should check into the hotel room and decide once we were settled. What did ya know? There was a Caribou Coffee and a Jimmy John's in the lobby of our hotel. They just became my "go-to" hotel if I ever need to stay overnight again. We checked in, got our food, and went straight to our room. I don't think I have eaten a sub faster in my life! Now the waiting game. When were these side effects going to kick in?

I ended up taking a short nap around 7:30 and woke up to the thickening saliva again...Yuck! I had an extra ginger ale from the hospital, which helped a bit, but the syrup in the soda almost made it worse. I'm thinking next time I will go for seltzer water. Sarah was amazing and ran down to the coffee shop for a Turtle Mocha (yummy), which really helped to get the gross taste out of my mouth, but it also kept me up until 4:00 am. But through it all, no side effects came.

There was nothing different from the previous treatment. HALLELUJAH! The next morning, we ate breakfast, took another morning nap, and checked out of the hotel.

Now, for the next part of my journey... a wig! I decided that I wanted to be prepared if and when this would happen, so we went to try some on. I really didn't know how I was going to react. I kind of thought I might just break down and cry in the middle of the whole process. But you know what? God was with me and gave me strength. It was actually fun; it was like getting your hair cut and colored over and over. Wendy, the sales associate, was amazing! She helped me try on a bunch of wigs and let us take pictures of them so I could take a few days to decide. Wigs are not a cheap thing either. Starting out at $150 and going up all the way to $500, and we are talking synthetic, not even real hair. I have a prescription for the wig, but I have to buy it myself and then send the receipt to my insurance company to be reimbursed (70% of it anyway). So I have a lot to think about with my choices, and I even bought a new hat that I will be able to wear as well. So even though I could have headed home Friday night and not spent the money on the hotel room, it was nice to have the peace of mind and to get to have a mini-vacation with the best LIL SIS in the WORLD!!!!!

By the time I dropped Sarah off and got back home and had dinner, it was almost 5:00 pm, and even though I hadn't really slept that much, I really couldn't take a nap. My sleep schedule really would have been off. So I stayed up but just hung out on the couch. By 8:00 pm, I was passed out, and I didn't wake up until 9:00 the next morning. That has not happened in years! During the last two treatments, my appetite had been off while I was on the pump and a few days after. Instead of following the clean eating, I began craving and was only able to eat what sounded good to me, which was a lot of processed foods. Thinking that at least I am eating was my mentality, and I let myself eat whatever I could get down. But this time was different. I made sure I had plenty of clean meals prepared before I even started treatment, and all day Sunday, I ate clean meals and snacks. I even got a good amount of ice water :) down too. I stayed on the couch most of the day and ate a lot of small meals and snacks, as I still had that gross taste in my mouth. I took a short nap and was asleep in bed by 10:00 pm. This morning when I woke up, I had a ton of energy and felt great. I truly believe that it was all the clean foods I had to eat the day prior, and I was even able to keep that going today at work. I packed some meals and snacks, and they kept me energized most of the day (we did have thirteen three-year-olds today). There are few things that can keep you energized for nine hours through that much excitement, but I wouldn't change it for the world. So now here I am writing this huge update, which I really didn't think was going to be this long, and listening to my "Lord of the Rings" station on Pandora. This girl is ready for bed and can't wait for what tomorrow brings. It will definitely bring a trip to the gym after work and another exciting day in the lives of three-year-olds!

Here is my little bit of inspiration for you tonight: "You never know how strong you are until being strong is the only choice you have."

All my Love,
Christine

wigging out

Another two weeks have gone by, and another round has been completed. I just finished my fourteenth round of chemo today, and I am still feeling great! I had an in-depth blood test on Thursday before chemo because my doctor wanted more information on my nutritional levels. This was a very early blood draw at 6:30 am because I was unable to eat after seven the night before and was only allowed eight ounces of water after midnight. I swear I am hypoglycemic because I get a little cranky when I'm "hangry" (a state of anger due to lack of food) Haha.

Once I got up to the chemo floor for my blood draw, they informed me that I either had to wait until 7:00 am to get my port accessed there or I could go to a different building to have it accessed right away. I asked if they could just do the blood test without accessing my port, and she agreed! Hallelujah! Thank goodness for a fast blood draw, cause as soon as it was done, I made a beeline for some food.

Once we got some food in our bellies (Sarah felt bad eating in front of me, so she was pretty hungry too), we made it up to my next appointment, where Sarah proceeded to take a nap. She can really sleep anywhere. I was excited to see Nurse Jessica; she is the one I see every time I go to Rochester, and she goes over my case with my oncologist before she meets me. So when I talk about meeting up with my doctor, it is her that I am actually seeing. She was excited to see my lab results and was very impressed with my NORMAL levels. She said that she couldn't believe how great my levels were and that just by looking at the labs, she would never believe that I was starting my fourteenth round of chemo. She asked me about the side effects that were common with the new drug, and I didn't have a single one. Even the hair thinning hasn't started. She was so surprised and happy that I am doing so well. She had given me the full dose of the new drug, and she had been worried about how I was going to tolerate it. Fourteen rounds is a lot of treatments, but one of the ways that cancer is smart is that it will become immune to the chemo drugs, and soon they will stop working (most likely what happened to the last drug and why I had a reaction to it).

Because my body has been doing so well with the drugs and the cancer is responding to the treatments, she wants to keep me going for at least another two to four rounds. I already have the next two rounds (May 29 and June 19) scheduled, with a CT scan scheduled on June 19th. The next two rounds are actually three weeks apart as opposed to two weeks due to my vacation to Colorado over Memorial Day weekend for my nephew's wedding. She gave me a quick physical and was happy to not find anything of concern. My lungs are clear, my liver and kidneys are normal-sized, and I have no swelling in my legs. Sometimes I think she gets worried when she can't find anything wrong. Haha. It was a pretty short visit as it was early in the day, and she has lots of patients to see.

Sarah and I had over four hours to kill before chemo started, so we went to try on some wigs again. After the last visit, the more I looked at the pictures we took, the less and less I liked them. I think it was because my actual hair has thinned so much that a short wig with lots of volume just didn't look right. So, I tried on wigs that were chin-length to shoulder-length. While trying them on, I felt like I was in an episode of "Say Yes to the Dress," but I referred to it as "Say Yes to the Wig," and I found one I really liked! I have a prescription for the wig, and after calling my insurance company, they told me that they would cover a portion of the wig, but I first need to purchase it, and then I can send in my claim and get reimbursed for the portion they cover. With the wig and everything I need to purchase for it (shampoo, conditioner, combs, stands, detangler, etc.) it will cost me over $500. I have set up a GoFundMe campaign for anyone who would like to help me with this purchase. I am very happy that I am not in need of it quite yet, but I am anxious to get it for when the thinning progresses.

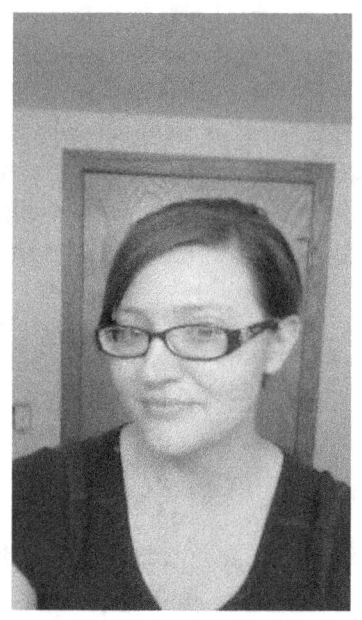

Sarah and I ran some errands and got some lunch before we returned to the hospital for chemo. I had to be given a dose of Atropine to stop the stomach cramps, runny nose, and thick saliva that come with the new chemo drug, but I was given it too early, and it began to wear off before I was done with my infusion. So, I was given another dose before I was done. I was able to take a little nap during treatment and finished it up with no other side effects. Last time I took a short nap in the evening and then was up until 4:00 am. This time, I slept from 2:30-3:00 am and then from five to six. It wasn't until I woke up Friday morning that I remembered the other use for Atropine; it's used to jump-start your heart. This may be the reason I have trouble sleeping.

Friday was cleaning day at my childcare center, and I wanted to be able to work part of the day to help out as well and use as little PTO as I could. I made it in by 9:00 am because I was a little jittery from the Atropine. I was able to work the rest of the day and still felt great when I left work.

I made a stop at the library to pick up some books I had on hold, and by the time I left, I was super tired. Once I got home, I ate some food and fell straight asleep on the couch. I proceeded to sleep on and off until 7:30 this morning. Today I got my haircut and had lunch with Kate. It was beautiful out, and it was nice to get out of the house. I spent the rest of the afternoon looking up clean eating recipes and planning out the next week of meals and snacks. I really do feel that my healthy eating and the vitamins I have been taking are a main reason that I still have a good amount of hair left. Kara, my hairdresser, said that if she had never cut my hair before today that she would have assumed I had a normal amount of hair, but because she has been cutting my super thick hair over the last six years that she could tell it had thinned. Thank you to all who have sent me head scarves, hats, and other little gifts to make this next transition a little easier. It is greatly appreciated.

I still get worried when I think about myself having no hair (like at the gym, or even at home looking into the mirror), but then I remember that I have so many family and friends by my side and that God will always be there for me to give me strength and courage. My trust and faith in God are what get me out of bed each day and to go on with my life. Cancer is such a scary topic, and it's even scarier when you are told that you have it. But playing the "What if" game or asking "Why me?" is not going to get you anywhere but depressed. I don't need to know why I got it... it doesn't change my outcome. I still have this fight, whether I understand it or not, and I choose to push through this fight and use everything I have in my power to overcome it!

All my Love,
Christine

god only gives you as much as you can handle

JUN. 3, 2015

I can't believe that it has been almost a month since my last journal entry. A lot has been going on, and I have been so busy that I apologize for the lack of information. At the end of May, I had a little vacation over Memorial Day weekend for my nephew's wedding. Yes, you heard me right—my NEPHEW'S wedding. And it wasn't even my eldest nephew (who just graduated fromCOLLEGE!!), and we celebrated that as well that weekend; it was my twenty-year-old nephew Josh and his new awesome wife, Megan! It was pretty fun seeing the looks as their friends asked how I had met the groom, and I would respond, "at his birth." It was even worse for Sarah, as she and my eldest nephew are only thirteen months apart. It was truly amazing out there, and I almost didn't want to come back. Haha.

The mountains are amazingly beautiful, and I can't wait to go back and visit. It was really nice to get together with the family and have some time just to hang out. Sarah and I flew back Tuesday night and didn't get into Eau Claire until 2:00 am Wednesday (I had to be at work at 8:00 am... bring on the coffee!) So, after that amazing vacation, it was time to return to work and see all "my kids." It's funny how just a few days away from them makes it feel so much longer. I woke up with a rather good amount of energy for only a few hours of sleep! But I also woke up to a text from the person I have been staying with that I needed to move out of the house by June 15th. That will snap you back into reality real fast! So, the last week has been packing, trying to find an apartment, working, getting utilities worked out, and oh yeah... treatment! I know God only gives us what we can handle, and if I can make it through this, y'all better watch out, 'cause nothing can take me down. It has been a very emotional and stressful week, but it has again opened my eyes to everyone around me who cares and supports me!

So now for the treatment update... round fifteen!!!!

So, my dad went with me for my treatment and to meet with the doctor. This was the first time that he had met anyone on my care team, so I was really glad when he was able to come. If you know me, which most of you do, I like to joke around. Well, when I realized I had a hat in my bag, I put it on and stuffed my hair underneath it (which I still have all of) and proceeded into my doctor's office. When she came in, she had an odd look on her face as she had never seen me with a hat on. She asked me how I was doing, and I told her that my hair looked a little different from before (not a lie, seeing as I had gotten it cut). She took a deep breath and asked to see what was going on under the hat. I whipped that hat off and said, "BUH BAM! It's still all there!" You should have seen the look on her face. We all started laughing, and then she went into her usual "well, just keep in mind that it most likely will start to thin the more you are on the drug." Well, right now it hasn't, and I am going to keep doing what I'm doing and praying to God it stays that way. She went over my lab results... NORMAL. I feel like I could almost copy and paste my doctor visit updates. I'm happy to hear the same thing each time! My white blood counts are a high normal (low is bad), but I have a cough, and she thinks that my body is just trying to fight it. She was worried that I was starting a sinus or respiratory infection and wanted to start me on antibiotics. Seeing as I vetoed her the last time, she wanted to put me on them. I let her go this time. I can count on one hand the number of times I have been on antibiotics in my life, so I knew I didn't need to worry about becoming immune to them or anything. She was very surprised that the last time I was on antibiotics was in seventh grade. I told her that until recently, I had been a very healthy person. Haha. Well, I have taken all my antibiotics, and they did nothing; I still have my cough. Go figure. I guess my body will take care of it! She gave me a quick physical and listened to my lungs, which were clear even though I had a cough, and said everything looked good. Somehow, we had gotten on the topic of my cake decorating, and I showed her some of the ones I had on my phone... she subtly told me her birthday was in September. :) She always asks the person I bring with if they have any questions or concerns. Dad said he was just so happy that I transferred my care down to Rochester. She said that usually they are fine with patients carrying out their treatment plans closer to home and only seeing them every few months for consults and scans, but when they found out the treatment plan that I had been on, they knew that I needed to have my primary care be with them. I couldn't agree more! It's hard to put your life in someone else's hands, and I know that my entire care team in Rochester is looking out for me! After the doctor's visit, I went for treatment, and who do you think was my neighbor? Ellis! I have mentioned Ellis in a previous post about how she is my inspiration anytime I get down. Knowing that this three-year-old is going through the same thing as me and usually with a HUGE smile makes me buck up and put my big girl pants on.

Ellis is also in my classroom at school, and she finds it so cool that we both have ports! If you haven't been to Rochester, it's HUGE! There are multiple buildings and multiple floors that one can receive treatment on, so the fact that she and I were in the same building, on the same floor, and across the hall from each other was a miracle. If you have ever been a teacher or a childcare provider and saw one of your kids outside of school, you get the look. It's the look of... "why are you not at school?" Well, you should have seen the look that I got from her. I was hooked up to my machine and covered in blankets. She was really shy at first, but that didn't last long. She had gone to her room to get set up, and I had fallen asleep. I think I blew her mind when she came back to see me and saw I was taking a nap! Her treatment wasn't as long as mine, so she came and saw me on the way out. She climbed up into the chair with me as her mom and dad talked with me and my dad. It was such a great experience to be able to show her that she isn't alone in this. I was actually wearing my "No one fights alone" bracelets, and she asked me why I had so many on. I told her that each one was for someone I knew, and I went through them, telling her each person they represented. When I got to orange (leukemia), I told her that it was for her. She looked up at me and just smiled.

It's been a crazy month, and I know the next month will be even crazier! So far, my next treatment is on June 19th, and I will be having a CT scan. So, lots of prayers for positive results! I will try my hardest to keep everyone updated on where I land, but for now, I will give you my dad's address if you need to get a hold of me. Thank you, everyone, for your love and support!

All my Love,
Christine

enjoying the little things!

JUN. 14, 2015

What a couple of weeks it has been! So, I am all moved out of my previous residence and have moved in with my grandma until I am able to find a new apartment. However, we just found out that she is allergic to my CAT, so I'm now looking for a temporary home for him until I can get into a new apartment. Life definitely has not been dull. And I am also looking for a second job to help pay for said apartment. I have been a pretty busy bee lately, and am currently house/dog sitting for a friend. It's nice to be back in the Chippewa country life. I really have missed it!

Treatment has still been going great. My next one is on Friday, and I will also be having a CT scan to know how the new drug is working. Lots of prayers and positive thoughts over the next week. I have been stressed out a lot since I got back from moving and trying to find a place for the animals, not to mention still working forty hours a week. But today at Mass, it was all about trusting in God and that He will deliver. Time to practice what I preach and just make the best out of today. God will provide! Just a short one today, as I will update you all on Friday about the latest scan.

All my Love,
Christine

nothing but good news!

JUN. 23, 2015

Round sixteen! My second set of eight rounds has now been completed.

On Friday, Sarah and I went to Rochester for round sixteen and a CT scan. My normal doctor was out of town, so yet again, I had to meet with a different oncologist on my care team. I think I have one more to see, and I've collected the whole set! Haha. Anyway, we made it down there at 6:30 am and got right in, which never happens. Actually, all my appointments that day were within five minutes of their scheduled times. So we go into the doctor's office to wait, and my nurse practitioner's nurse (following me?) came in to find Sarah lying across the couch and me lying on the examination table. She had a look of dread on her face as she entered. "Everything okay?" she asked.

"Yep, just really tired," I said.

"Oh, thank God. I thought someone was sick."

"Well, I am in the oncologist's office." Haha. So we talked about symptoms over the last three weeks, and moving, and manicures/pedicures. Pretty much had a girls' talk for fifteen minutes. Allison knows Sarah and me. She knows we are crazy, and we don't dwell on what we can't change. However, my fill-in oncologist does not. She comes in with a serious face and tone and introduces herself. She asks a few questions and then proceeds to the scans. Now this is what I've been waiting for. Lay it on me!

"The scans are good!"

Hallelujah, praise Jesus! She pulled up the section of my liver and said that she actually had trouble finding the mass on the new scan. What she didn't know is that there used to be two! Amazing! She pulled up my lungs, and some of the masses were even half the size as before. I couldn't believe it. She pulled up my labs, and everything was... say it with me... normal! Then she showed me my CEA level. That is the level of cancer cells in your blood. Even a person without cancer can have a level under three and still be considered normal. Now, just to put this into perspective, my CEA level ten months ago was 25.9! Today, it is 1.4! One Point Four! I could not believe it. Cut in half again. God is truly amazing and shows me every day that He loves me. I have had a very sucky month, but I wouldn't trade it for anything to be able to live where I am supported and loved, to not be in fear, and to learn that God will never abandon me. I find it funny that this has been an extremely stressful month, but nothing to do with my health has stressed me. "Don't take life too seriously... you'll never get out alive!"

All my Love,
Christine

light at the end of the tunnel

JUL. 11, 2015

Round seventeen is underway, and I am excited to share the news from my latest doctor's appointment. Sarah and I traveled once again down to Rochester for labs, a doctor's consult, and chemo. There is always a pretty long wait between the blood draw for labs and the doctor's visit, so Sarah got an hour nap, and I worked on my training for my second job as a Jamberry consultant. I have been looking for a flexible second job, and this just seemed to fit all the criteria I needed. I had been waiting for almost a month to hear whether my disability claim was going to be approved or denied. Well, I finally got a hold of the caseworker they assigned me, and after a five-minute conversation, I was told that I made too much money to qualify, but if I ever go down to part-time, that I can reapply. Well, that's not going to happen anytime soon, and I'm guessing with my new second job that really isn't going to happen. I was pretty upset after the phone call because with missing days for treatment, I already take a big enough hit in my paycheck. Then to find out that my paycheck never got deposited because of a fluke in the system. Needless to say, my blood pressure was

134/72, which isn't bad, but it hasn't been over 115/64 in the last eight months.

So, onto the big enchilada... oh man, that sounds really good right now... the doctor's visit! So once again, I call her my doctor, but she is technically a nurse practitioner... she's my middleman to the oncologist. She took a look at my CT scan from the previous visit (I had a fill-in because she was at a conference, and thank God she went to it—I will tell you why in a minute), and she was very pleased with the results. As some of you know, I was done with phase 2 of the treatment plan... Man; I sound like a science experiment. "Now commencing phase 3. Phase 3 is a go!" So, the next phase of my treatment plan will be four more rounds of the traditional chemo that I have been receiving. There was previous talk of giving my body a break after the second set of eight rounds, but the way I look at it is my body is strong and stubborn, you wouldn't be giving my body a break, you would be giving the cancer a break, and I'm not down with that! So after four more rounds two weeks apart (two months), I will be moving to "chemo-lite." Like the name? "Chemo-lite" will be going down to Rochester for labs, a doctor's visit, and one—count them—one chemo drug that takes ten minutes to administer! After that, I will take pills for three weeks that are my chemo drugs. Sorry, Larry, you and I won't be seeing each other too much after that! It is a long way to drive, but I love everyone in Rochester, and feel I get the best care there plus I love my doctor's visits. Jessica (NP AKA DR) actually said her face hurt from laughing so much during our visit. I bet that doesn't happen too often in her day. Now for the exciting part... are you ready? Jessica wants to schedule me for another lung biopsy in the near future (six to nine months) after my rounds of chemo are done, as I cannot be on Avastin (ten-min chemo drug) as it causes bleeding. The reason I need another biopsy is that there is not enough tissue left to test a new treatment on. She wants more fresh tissue (I just got a zombie movie flashback typing that, Haha) to test this new therapy that she heard about at the conference she attended. If it reacts well, it will be "phase 4." Now I am giving you her exact quote she told us, "I'm not going to say CURE (as a smile crept on her face) but I'm going to say it's been making it go away!"

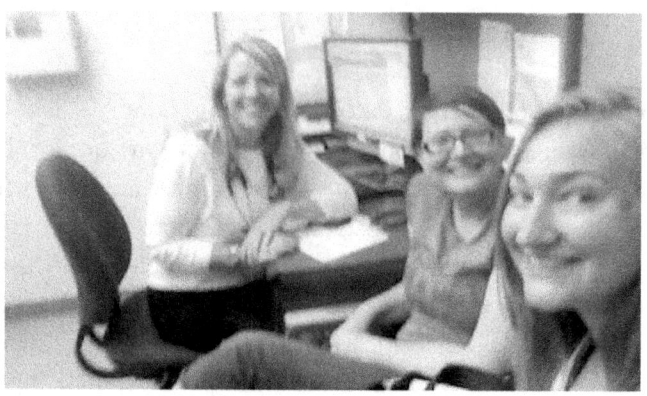

How AMAZINGLY AWESOME IS THAT?!? She said I am a prime candidate for it as I am young, active, and tolerating my current treatment extremely well. She is still baffled by the fact that I still have my hair! And as long as I make it through my next three rounds, and the one I'm on with my hair, I most likely won't lose it once I go to "chemo-lite!" More great news. Chemo went fine. I did more training and watched Shark Week, but the cherry on the cake was that I got a call back about a FREE massage on Sunday for cancer patients. I will be having a fifty-minute massage tomorrow for nothing (well, I still plan on tipping the masseuse). And my pump is scheduled to come off thirty minutes before my appointment! I am so excited! I haven't had a massage in over three years, and I miss them so much! So, it was a great trip to Rochester.

On the way back, I decided I was going to start writing a book about my journey and how staying positive through this journey has benefited me and those around me. I may be asking some of you in the future about using quotes or comments you have sent me or posted on the CaringBridge page, so keep them coming! Your prayers and positive thoughts are definitely working, and I am so thankful for them.

All my Love,
Christine

the only "c" word i want to hear!

JUL. 25, 2015

Round eighteen... I'm actually losing count. Haha.

So, another trip to Rochester has been completed, and I am happy to report that I once again received good and hopeful news. I started out with the usual blood draw, and the results were all NORMAL! But I'm sure you all were expecting that. So onto the doctor's visit with Dr. Jessica (and I found out I can call her that even though her title is nurse practitioner). So anyway... I was her first patient of the day, so I got into all my appointments right on time or early! We went over the blood tests, and she gave me the okay to start round eighteen of treatment. I had wanted more in-depth information on my treatment plan because there were some areas I was assuming they would go a certain way, and I wanted to make sure we were on the same page. So here is the OFFICIAL treatment plan as it stands now. I have two more rounds after this one of regular-Larry-toting treatment (as in Rochester for two chemo drugs followed by wearing a pump for two days). I love you, Larry. You 're saving my life, but I think we need a break! So, on August 21, I will be having a CT scan. Depending on what is found on the scan, she will decide if she wants to do the lung biopsy at that time or wait for the following CT scan after "chemo-lite." I responded that if she waits too long, there may not be anything to biopsy! She hopes this is the case. "Chemo-lite" will be going to Rochester for anti-nausea meds and Avastin. Which will cut my treatment time from three hours to thirty minutes! Then, I will take a low-dose pill of my current chemo drugs for three weeks. Right now, I am on the maximum dose she can give me of my chemo drugs, but they don't hang around for the full two weeks at full-strength. So, now I will have a current supply of cancer-killing machines in my body! After the three weeks are up, I will be heading back down to Rochester to do it all again! I will do four rounds of "chemo-lite" and then have another CT scan. Once it has been decided when I will be having the lung biopsy (one month or four months from now), I will be taken off Avastin (the drug that finds cells with too many blood vessels attached aka chemo cells, and it destroys the surrounding blood vessels turning off the cancer cell's blood supply... BYE BYE), as it does cause bleeding which would not be good for a lung biopsy. The lung biopsy is so that they can do a full genetic workup of my cancer to find the genetic marker that the new drug she wants to try reacts to. This genetic marker has been found a lot in younger patients (lots of prayers will be needed for me to have this specific marker!). There are two new drugs that she feels I am a PRIME candidate for, but the one she wants most to try is the one I will be genetically tested for. It's so new that the FDA hasn't even cleared it yet, and it is still in a trial state. If I get on this drug, and it is approved... hello medical journals! Haha. She then said, "People have been CURED on this drug!" (That's the C word I wanted to hear. LOL). So, that is the official treatment plan.

Let me just update you on what Sarah is doing at the time of this conversation... sleeping on the couch with her head on my lap, and snoring. Haha. She has been such a trooper with all these early morning appointments.

The next one on August 7th isn't until 10:00 am, but the following one with the CT scan is at 7:00 am... I think we will drive down the night before and get a hotel room. So, back to the doctor's visit. My doctor had asked me if I ever thought about what could happen with the diagnoses I have. Doc, if I haven't fallen apart yet, almost a year later, it's gonna take a lot to break me down! And I have thought about the possible outcomes. I know I could die from this, and I know with the odds I have been given that I have a better chance of dying than surviving, but I'm not dwelling on it. A doctor could take the odds of fatal car accidents and tell me that in the next ten years, I will most likely die in a car accident. That isn't going to stop me from driving every day. I plan for the future and worry about today. I told her, "I'm not dying today of cancer or tomorrow, and that's as far as my worries go."

Then we got on the topic of the book I am going to write. When I told her the title **"How Cancer Improved My Life,"** the look on her face was priceless!

"You want to name it what?" she asked.

I repeated it.

"Okay," she said. "How has cancer improved your life?" she asked.

Oh....let me count the ways.

1. I am closer to everyone in my family—parents, siblings, aunts, uncles, grandma, you name it! I have an amazing support staff.

2. I am closer to God. I no longer go to church out of guilt of being a bad Christian, but because it makes me happy and I enjoy going.

3. I no longer feel the fear of what people think about me, what people are saying about me, etc. This is my life, and the only opinion about me that matters is mine!

4. I was able to look back at my relationships with ex-boyfriends and realized that I knew they were done way before they ended, but I was too afraid to leave out of fear of what I would do next.

5. I have a much higher quality of life now, and I am more positive, kind, friendly, happy, and outgoing than before. Plus, I am not in constant pain like I was before I was diagnosed.

She sat there for a minute and said, "You need to write this book. I have so many young patients who ask me if there is anyone they can talk to who is their age and is going through or has beaten this."

I grabbed my business card from my wallet and slid it across the desk. "My email, phone number, and my CaringBridge are my name and are public. If you have anyone that you feel will benefit from talking to me, I give you my permission to give out my number."

She looked up at me and said two little words: "You're amazing."

I know the fear of being so young and diagnosed with such an advanced cancer. If anyone is in my shoes (diagnosed with colorectal cancer at a young age, at any stage), please take this advice... DO NO RESEARCH YOUR CANCER for at least three to six months after your initial diagnosis! You will become overwhelmed, and the odds/percentages/prognoses are years of numbers and cases from patients in their 70s, 80s, and even 90s. These numbers do not apply to us!

Make your own odds! I was told I have a 10% chance of being cancer-free, and you best believe I am making it into that 10%. The more of us that do, the more we will increase that number tenfold! Believe in YOU! You got this!

Okay, back to the book (sorry, this is such a long entry, but I feel especially inspired today!) So, there are going to be people who read the name of my book and want to slap me in the face. Before you do, read the first chapter. This book is not just for people diagnosed with cancer or any type of disease. I want this book to inspire people of all walks of life to see what positivity and support can do to a person's life. I truly believe that you are the only person who can make yourself happy. This is a one-day-at-a-time habit to incorporate into your life. One of my favorite quotes says, "You don't know the strength you have until it is your only option." I remember reading a friend's post about being diagnosed with breast cancer (this was months before I was diagnosed), and her positive behavior radiated from her Facebook posts. I could tell her mood and attitude from the way she spoke, and I remember thinking, "There is no way I could be that positive if I were diagnosed with cancer." Lo-and-behold, a few months down the road, I too was given the choice of giving up or powering through! And like my friend, I chose to power through. I am happy to report that my friend is now CANCER-FREE! I feel that being positive in a situation like I am in is a huge factor in why I am able to power through. And some may disagree with me. I know that people who have watched a family member suffer through cancer, even though they were positive, and they may think I am full of it. But just like rubbing a penny for luck, being positive in your life can't hurt, so why not try it!

Okay, I have gone on long enough, so I will leave you with one more tidbit, and then I promise I am done. I have NEVER seen the same patient twice during chemo, and yesterday I saw Ellis again, and she was once again right across the hall from me. I don't know if it helps her to see me doing the same thing as she does, but seeing her smiling face definitely helps me! Nice call, God!

All my Love,
Christine

the big 3-0!

JUL. 30, 2015

It's heeeeerrrreeeee! (Think *Poltergeist*), I am now officially a thirty-year-old! And it wasn't anything like I expected!

After a huge group discussion over whether we were going to make ice cream or lemonade, my three-year-olds at work decided that it was definitely going to be lemonade! I'm down for that! So, I headed to work this morning with coffee and lemons on my mind! After a free coffee for my birthday (the best kind), and a trip to the store for lemons, popsicles, and cheese crackers, I headed off to work. I was greeted by many coworkers, children, and parents with lots of birthday wishes. We made our lemonade, of course, from scratch; it has to be educational, too. Haha. Each child got to help squeeze the lemons and then asked if they could eat them. Really? You want to eat the lemons? Go for it! Best birthday present I could ask for. You should have seen those puckered-up faces!

A child in my class had invited his grandma to read us a story today. It turns out that I knew his grandma from back when my parents had done Amway! Turns out, this child, who has been in my class for the last two months, is the child of a friend I had when I was six years old! And to add a cherry on the cake... it is her birthday today, too! MIND BLOWN! I couldn't believe it. Someone whom I had not seen in almost twenty-five years was now a parent of a child in my class! Way to go, God!

I was able to leave work early, but found out that my dinner plans with Sarah were canceled as she had come down with the stomach flu! I had asked a few people if they were free for dinner, but to no avail. I wasn't able to secure a replacement. Sarah and I had planned to get sushi, and I had really been looking forward to going. Finally, I decided that I was going to dinner with myself! I have only done this once before, and I always find it a little uncomfortable. But I am thirty now, and I should be able to have dinner solo if I want to! So, I went to the restaurant and sat at the sushi counter. I had been there a few times with Sarah, and the chef I had tonight was the one we always got! It was slow in the restaurant, so she talked with me as she made my delicious sushi rolls. I had brought a notebook to start the writing process, but I ended up putting it away and just enjoyed the time I was having. I never once thought about how I looked eating alone or what others might be think-ing. I just talked with the chef and enjoyed the simple things in life... like a caterpillar roll! Oh, calm down; there aren't any actual caterpillars in it! So, I finished my three rolls (nowhere near Sarah's record of six) and headed home.

As I drove with the windows down and the warm summer breeze running through my hair, I was thankful. I had experienced yet another area of my life that had been improved by cancer. FEAR. As I thought about being single on such a "monumental" birthday, I looked back on my life and asked myself the question... Would I rather be single with an amazing support system of friends and family? Or would I rather be in a toxic relationship that I know will never work out and isn't good for me? Single and supported! I've spent so many years in relationships that I knew they were never going to change because I was afraid of being by myself. This journey has opened my eyes to so many aspects of my life, and I have finally found so much clarity with issues that have confused me for so long. I am thankful to you, who are reading this; I am thankful for every single person who wished me a happy birthday; and I am thankful for another year of life that isn't always promised! Oh, and the icing on this birthday cake? My fortune from dinner... "You will live a long life but never be old!"

All my Love,
    Christine

so much for no excitement!

L ast Sunday, I took off my pump and was in a bit of a hurry as I was heading to our Schrader Family Gathering. Well, I didn't clamp the tubing right and ended up losing all the solution that stayed in my port tubing. The solution is in there so that blood cannot clot in the tubing and cause blood clots. I called urgent care to see if I would need to come in to get a new tube of solution or if it would be okay to leave until my next appointment in two weeks. I talked to a nurse at Mayo Eau Claire, and she told me that she would have the on-call oncologist call me in the next twenty minutes. Seeing as I live less than five minutes away, Sarah and I drove there just in case. As soon as we walked in, I got a call from the oncologist to let me know that I didn't need a new solution, and it would be fine to wait the two weeks. So, I went home, took off my pump, and headed to the party.

I had felt pretty run down Friday... and Saturday... and Sunday was showing to be the same. It wasn't that I was tired; I just had no energy to do anything. As Sunday went on, I kept thinking that it didn't make sense that I wouldn't need new solution in my port. I mean, blood clots are not a good thing to have in your body. So, on Monday afternoon, I called Mayo Rochester to talk to my doctor and get a second opinion. After talking to a nurse, she told me that she couldn't say that my waiting two weeks would be okay. It might be fine, but she couldn't say for certain. She put me on hold to ask around, and when she came back, she still had the same answer. So, I asked if I should just play it safe and get it flushed with new solution. You could almost hear the relief in her voice when she told me yes, and that if I was close, I could come down and get it done. I told her I lived in Eau Claire, and that I would call Mayo Eau Claire to see if they could get me in. I called them, and they couldn't get me in until today at two. So, I went on my lunch break and was actually pretty excited because I hadn't seen the nurses for the last seven months. The flush went fine, and my port was working great. That alone gave me peace of mind... I would have worried for the next two weeks, hoping it was okay.

So, I saw my old nurses, and they couldn't believe how well I looked. They were asking how I had been doing, and I told them I had just finished round nineteen. They were all astonished and asked if I was getting treatment in Rochester. I kinda felt like I was cheating on my hairdresser. I can't believe I have already had eleven rounds in Rochester. I had been toying with the idea of getting treatment back in Eau Claire once I moved to "chemo-lite," but the fact that an oncologist in Eau Claire told me it was fine to wait, and a nurse in Rochester wasn't okay with me waiting shows me that Rochester is the place to be. Yeah, the two-hour drive there and back for a ten-minute treatment isn't ideal, but this is my life, and I will do whatever it takes to live it!

All my Love,
    Christine

happy one-year anniversary!

AUG. 24, 2015

Thursday, August 20th, was my first anniversary of <u>Fighting Like a Beast</u>!

It is crazy how much has changed and gone on over the last year. Last Thursday, I spent the day at work, and we had a field trip to Irvine Park, where we had lunch and went on a treasure hunt, as it was Pirate Week at school. The kids all had a great time, and we found our treasure (plastic gold coins in a treasure chest lunchbox). But man, were they excited! There were four other daycare centers there, and as it should happen, I had worked for two of them and knew a lot of the teachers of the third, as I worked with them over the last few years.

As I was watching the children in my class play on the jungle gym, a little boy from a different center caught my eye. I took a second glance and realized it was the nephew of an ex-boyfriend. I had been there when he was born and had watched him quite a bit his first year of life. I instantly started to tear up and wasn't able to see him again as the center had left shortly after. I was glad that I got to see how much he had already grown and was happy for the "Blast from the Past" moment. It made me realize how far I had come in the few years.

Well, we finished playing and had our lunch, and soon it was time to get on the bus, which I was glad for as it wasn't very warm. While walking to the bus with twelve three-year-olds in tow, I heard my name being shouted, and who do you think it was? My bestie, Kate! Which is funny because I was going to see if she wanted to join us at the park, but never got around to it. So, I got to talk with her for a few minutes before we headed back to the center. The ride back to the center went fine, but you could tell it was rest time, and the kids were tired. I was happy to get back as well because I was still cold from the park. After we got back and settled, I noticed that I was still unable to warm up, and then it happened. That chill you get when you aren't cold but have a fever. Uh oh! Fevers and treatment don't go together. It was time for my break, and I went and checked my temperature... 100.3 degrees. Not horrible —but not good. I had to call my doctor if my temp goes over 100.5 degrees. So, I finished my break and headed back to my room. I let the other teacher go on her break and threw on another sweater, but was still chilled. An hour later, she came back, and I went and checked it again.... 100.9 degrees. Okay, now it's officially a problem. So, I helped with snacks and getting the kids ready to go outside, and then left work for the day.

I immediately called my doctor in Rochester and waited for a call back. I was almost home when I got the call from Allison, Dr. Jessica's head nurse. "You have to go to the ER," she told me.

Ummmmm....what? The ER as in emergency room, for a fever? This can't be right. It's a fever. I just need to go home and sleep. But I did it. I went to the ER and told them I was a chemotherapy patient with a fever of 101, and that I needed a blood draw. They had to check my counts to see if and where my infection was. So, I got there around four and waited to be looked at. They took my temp again, and now it was at 100.4 degrees. They took me back to a room and had me pee in a cup, took a blood sample and took a chest x-ray. And do you know what they found?!?! NOTHING! All labs were normal! Yep, that's me. Even with a fever, I have normal labs. So, they couldn't find the source of the fever and sent me home, but they made sure I knew that if my fever came back, I was to come back to the ER. It was now six o'clock, and I headed home. I'm not sure why, but when I get sick, I revert to my eight-year-old self. All I wanted was my dad's chicken noodle soup (which I had to compromise for my mom's quick fix of Mrs. Grass... but no Veg-All). Then, I put on my mom's old sweater, which I refer to as my "sick sweater" as I only wear it when I am sick, and watched Disney movies. And this is what happens every time I get sick! I ended up falling asleep by 8:30 pm and not waking up until 9:00 am the next morning. Well, after thirteen hours of sleep, I felt really good, and I didn't have a fever. But because I had had a fever the day prior, my treatment for round twenty was canceled and moved to this weekend. So, now I am due down in Rochester this Friday, and will hopefully be driving down the night before as my first appointment will be at 6:40 am!

I was really hoping that my last regular chemo round was going to be the day after my one-year anniversary, but it was nice to have the reminder of all that I have gone through and that I have made it this far. Sometimes, I can get lax with the precautions I take to make sure I stay healthy, and it was an eye-opener that even though I have done really well, I can still get sick, and that would complicate things a lot. So, back to being a germaphobe and making sure I am taking care of my body! Clean eating and exercise!!!!

All my Love,
Christine

you better get on living or dying

AUG. 29, 2015

Well, round twenty is in the works! I had a CT scan yesterday, and the results are great! The small mass on my liver hasn't changed at all, so she thinks it's not alive anymore because it's so small and light. So, it's just damaged tissue left over, kind of like scar tissue. She was able to find the second mass on my liver, but it's almost undetectable unless you know that it's there. The masses on my lungs has shrunk considerably as well. They have even started to show blackness in the middle of the masses, which means that they are dying from the inside out and are actually caving in on themselves. She was very impressed with my results—so impressed that she wants to do another two rounds of full chemo before they put me on chemo-lite. So, Larry will be hanging around a bit longer than expected. But with how I am responding to treatment and the few side effects I do have, she wants to push it out as much as she can. Funny that when I first started in Rochester, they were only going to do eight to ten more rounds (that would have made rounds sixteen to eighteen), and now I'm looking at full chemo rounds until round twenty-two! They underestimated my fighting capability and my stubbornness.

After going over the scans, she went over my labs, and the only thing out of the norm is my protein level, but with a week's worth of jaw pain due to my wisdom teeth and a week for the stomach flu, and then another week of allergies, I wasn't eating too much. And what I was eating wasn't always clean. So back to the clean diet and back to ALL normal test results!

I had brought up that it was my one-year anniversary last week, and she asked how I was feeling about it. The last year has been a struggle, but my life has improved. It feels weird to say that, but it's true. For the first three months, I was completely overwhelmed, and I couldn't process anything that wasn't happening that day or the next. I literally had to go a day at a time. Dr. Jessica asked if I still felt that way, and I told her no. She asked me how I feel now about everything. I feel optimistic that I will beat this and be cancer-free. In the beginning, there were so many areas that weren't defined. I didn't think I was going to get married, or have kids, or ever be truly happy... I didn't know how much time I had, or who would want to be in a relationship with something as huge as a cancer diagnosis.

Cancer is not a death sentence! It's a huge obstacle, and sometimes it doesn't end the way we want, but I'm not going to let it control my life. I was watching *The Shawshank Redemption* last night, which is one of my favorite movies. And a line in there stuck with me: "You better get busy living or get busy dying." I choose to live my life to the fullest of my ability. Again, thank you for all your support and love.

All my Love,
Christine

i am a fighter!

SEPT. 19, 2015

Well... I can't fall back asleep, so I might as well journal. Today was round twenty-two, and it went a lot better than the two previous rounds. It just so happens that my mom was in town and was able to go with me. She was a little nervous, as she had never gone to a treatment with me in Rochester... in fact, I don't know if she has ever been able to go to a treatment round.

Anyhooo... my doctor had the day off, so there was no doctor's visit today—just labs and chemo. But I got a bit of bad news in the billing area. I found out today that they are sending me to collections for a $2500 bill! Completely dumbfounded, I asked when I had been sent, as I had not received a letter saying I was to be sent. They sent me to collections on September 14, four days prior. When I asked when the first letter had been sent out. She told me on July 28th. Looks like ALL my mail was never forwarded from the Eleva address, and I didn't officially change it with Mayo until early August. Well, now that it's in collections, I can't apply for assistance from Mayo. My max out of pocket is $2000, so I wait until I hit my max out of pocket before I apply, so I don't have to apply twice. If I had actually received the notice, I would have done it right away. Not a great way to end my chemo visit, but I have lots of calls to make Monday morning to see what my options are. I just find it weird that I had one letter sent, they received no response, and I changed my address. And no one from Mayo even attempted to contact me via email or phone. Or... hello I'm there every other week, you could have asked to see me sooner. END RANT

Dwelling on the negative won't get me anywhere; it will get paid... eventually :) Back to chemo. The round went well, and I had a lot more energy than in the previous rounds. Seeing as my mom has never been to Rochester, we hit a few shops, and even went to dinner at Lake Hallie Bar and Grill, where my brother cooks. Gotta love Friday fish fry. It took me a bit to fall asleep, and I finally did at midnight only to wake up at 1:00 am, and so far, I am WIDE AWAKE!

Sarah and I have been looking for apartments, and hopefully will be moved into one of the ones we narrowed it down to by October, with the financial help from my mom and her husband. I'm excited to be reunited with Lucky! He's been living with Sarah since June. I'm sure Sarah will be happy to be done being a foster mom to him too. Haha.

All in all, things are going well, and I have still had very few side effects of what I could actually be experiencing. Mostly just fatigue and more hair thinning. But I only have one more full-strength round after this, and then I will get a break and go on maintenance. She's thinking three rounds, three weeks in between, and then another CT scan to see how I reacted. When on maintenance, it's such a low-dose that I most likely won't see any shrinking of masses, but hopefully it's a strong enough dose to keep them from growing. I will be doing lots of praying between now and then. Hopefully, she will have more info on when she wants to do the lung biopsy on the next visit... October 2 for those of you keeping track;)

All my Love,
Christine

be your own advocate!

OCT. 11, 2015

I t's been a pretty crazy couple of weeks, so I apologize for the late entry. Last Friday (October 2), I went to Rochester for what I was hoping was to start on chemo-lite. When I got to the doctor's office, I was actually seeing a different oncologist. My primary doctor, Dr. Jessica, was on vacation, so they scheduled me with a doctor on my care team. My appointment lasted fifteen minutes, and he only talked to me for five minutes of it. The rest was typing on the computer, and he actually left the room to take a page. At the end of it, he told me that I was going to have two more full rounds of chemo, and then we would set a CT scan, and IF he was happy with the results and there was no growth, then after round eleven, I could start on the pills.

HOLD UP!

He obviously didn't read my chart!

A. Because I started round fourteen that day, (round twenty-two total) not round eleven, and if he had looked at my previous scans, he would have seen that the only time I have ever had growth was when I was off chemo for two months at the be- ginning of the year!

B. THIS IS NOT THE PLAN! For those of you who don't know me, I'm pretty stubborn, and I don't like plans being changed without a reason I understand.

So, he sent me on my way, and I headed to chemo, but I was LIVID! I ended up crying to the nurse who was setting up my chemo, and right then and there, I wrote an email to Dr. Jessica. I told her I refused to see him again and would reschedule if he was the only one available. I finished chemo and went home for another weekend—too tired to leave the couch or my bed. It took me all day Saturday to muster up the energy to run to the store for food.

So, then Monday came around, and I headed back to work. It was a long week, and I don't know if it was the funk I was in from the bad doctor's appointment or what, but it took a lot to get through it. To add stress into the mix, I was trying to get approved for an apartment. I have been filling out forms and dropping off information for almost three weeks, and I was starting to get an uneasy feeling about it all.

By Thursday I was praying to God—something's gotta give. I remember repeating that in my head. It was all starting to pile on top of me, and I didn't know what to do to make it better.

Then Friday came... I was able to go home early, and when I left, I saw a text on my phone.

"Your application has been accepted."

I called the property manager, and he told me I could come in on Monday and sign the lease and start moving in right away! YAY! Finally, some good news. But it didn't stop there. A few minutes later my cell rang... it was Dr. Jessica! She called to see what all had happened at the appointment. I went over the details, and she apologized profusely. She said, "That never should have happened, and you need to know that it's you, me, and Grothey (my oncologist). The other doctor is just a fill-in. We are not changing your treatment plan." She went on to say that the last time she saw me, we had said four more rounds, and then chemo-lite. Sorry, doc! I love ya and all, but no, we didn't. I told her that I remembered her saying that we were having two more and then going on the pills. She checked her notes, and I was right—October 2 was supposed to be my last round. "Okay, I will move your scan to the sixteenth, and if everything looks good and there is no growth, we will start you on chemo-lite."

Hallelujah! Being stubborn pays off! Thank you, God! I know some of you who read this may not be very religious or believe in something different from what I do, and I'm not here to preach at you, but over and over I give my problems up to God, and He delivers. When life gets too big for me, I pray to Him, and He returns it with what I need, whether it's strength to get through the day, guidance to find my path, or energy to get out of bed. He has always been there for me, just like all of you and your amazing support!

All my Love,
Christine

happy halloween!

OCT. 31, 2015

It's been a while since I have posted, and that's because this month has been so crazy! Sarah and I moved into our new apartment on the fifteenth, and the next day we went down to see the doctor in Rochester. The CT scan looked good, and my labs were back to normal. She gave me the green light to start chemo-lite, and instead of my three-hour treatment, I had a fifteen-minute treatment and was scheduled to start pills a few days later. I would take the pills for two weeks, have a week off, and then go back down to Rochester.

We headed home with the understanding that I would get a call from the pharmacy with how much my copay would be for the pills, and then they would send them to my house. I did get the call from the pharmacy, but I certainly wasn't expecting what they told me. The two weeks were going to cost me $1000! Just for one dose. My max out of pocket for prescription drugs is $1000, so after the first dose, it would just be $25 each time after that. But after January 1st, it would start over, and once again, one dose would cost me $1000. I didn't fill the prescription and called my doctor on Monday. We came to an agreement that we would take a break from chemo until November 20th. On the 20th, I will go to Rochester, have a CT scan, and see the doctor. If everything looks good, then I will get another month off from chemo. If the doctor is concerned with my CT scan, then I will have a chemo-lite dose with the pump... which costs a lot less. I will still wear Larry for the two days and disconnect. If my scans stay as good as they have been, I could be off of chemo until next year! So, lots of prayers... from my understanding, if the masses don't grow, I will be considered "IN REMISSION."

So, my doctor scheduled me for a lung biopsy on November 6th, and we will find out if I am able to start the super new treatment. So, other than that, I don't really have too much going on. I have a seasonal job at Joann's to help with some bills... my goal is to be debt-free (except for my car) by the end of the year!

Sarah and I are enjoying our new apartment and have only had one "box fight" since we moved in (see my Facebook page for the video). Thank you all for your love and support through this journey!

All my Love,
  Christine

2016

2015 recap

I can't believe it's been so long since I last updated my CaringBridge. The holidays were super busy, as I'm sure all of yours were as well. So, I will give a little recap of what has happened these last few months.

November

I went back to Rochester for my lung biopsy on the sixth. It went extremely well, even better than my first one. I had no complications from it. Sarah went with me and was excited to record my coming off the drugs. When they wheeled me back to recovery, I had to go right by the waiting room. I'm lying flat on my back as they wheel me past, and as they do, I raise my hand straight in the air and start frantically waving at Sarah. I hear the whole waiting room start to giggle, and then Sarah goes, "Hi Christine." She came back and checked on me, phone at the ready for some awesome blackmail/YouTube video, but I wasn't really out of it. She talked with the nurse and asked her about it, and the nurse told her, "She didn't need as much medication as we normally give; she's a pretty tough cookie." They gave me medicine to calm me down and numb the area they were going to biopsy, but I had to stay coherent, so I could follow directions with my breathing. All said and done, the procedure went great, and we stayed overnight as a precaution. Two weeks later, I was back to see how the last six weeks had gone without any treatment. The CT scan and labs had shown that the masses in my lungs had started to regrow. So, chemo-lite was going to start that day. It's basically the same process; I just don't have one of my three drugs.

December

I continued with chemo-lite every two weeks. I was still working at Joann's part-time. Turns out my manager is a cancer survivor and had been really understanding with my treatment. Each round of treatment had gone well with few side effects. I had my sister, Sue Ann, and her family over for Christmas, and my mom had come up the week before. I rang in the New Year by falling asleep on the couch at 10:30 and rolling into bed a few minutes before midnight. Sarah and I spent all of New Year's Day binge-watching TV and coloring in my Harry Potter coloring book I got for Christmas. Haha. She told me I was not allowed to do ANYTHING all day. And I happily complied.

January

I have had one more round of chemo-lite and will go back to the doctor on January 29th for another consult. It's weird to say, but I'm ready to go back on full doses. That's the only way I'm going to beat cancer into submission, and I plan on doing that this year! It saddens my heart to know that we lost David Bowie and Alan Rickman this week, both to this horrible disease. Alan Rickman is one of my favorite actors, and I can't believe I won't be seeing him in movies anymore. I also lost a friend the day after Christmas. He's the father of a good friend and had only been diagnosed a month earlier with lung cancer. It went so fast, I am still in shock that he is gone. His funeral service was being held the same day I had treatment, so I hurried back to town and was able to pay my respects to an amazing man. I got to meet a lot of his amazing family and friends. He will be sorely missed. But I know he will be with me on the 29th as I go in for my twenty-seventh round of treatment.

Thank you to all who read and comment on my posts. I love hearing from you. The support and love you give me keep me going. I hope 2016 is an amazing year for you all!

All my Love,
Christine

it's the little things

JAN. 30, 2016

I am now on round twenty-seven, and it is going very well. This is another round of chemo-lite, so I don't have as many side effects. My hair has started to thicken, and is even long enough for pigtails. I have even been able to put in two French braids—it's the little things. Haha.

I talked with my doctor yesterday and told her I was ready to go back on full-dose chemo. She instantly asked, "Why? What happened?" with a concerned look on her face.

I told her nothing had changed, but I wasn't going to kick cancer's butt being on maintenance. I'm sure she doesn't have a lot of patients who request upping their chemo dosage. I am worried that I may lose my hair instead of it just thinning out, but I'm hoping for the same symptoms as the last time I was on it. Weird thing to be hopeful for. I am almost fully recovered from my ear infection

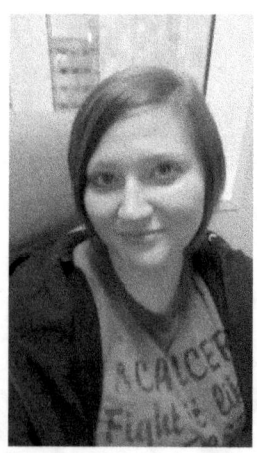

and still have normal blood labs with perfect blood pressure. So besides cancer, I'm in perfect health. :) I have still been going to the gym a few times a week and working full-time. I am really trying to keep to clean eating, and it has helped with my energy levels. All in all, I have been feeling really good and still feel hopeful for the future.

My next project, besides writing a book, is to become a peer support counselor for others fighting cancer, especially people my age. I'm really excited about this part of my journey and can't wait to begin.

I can't believe it's almost February. February 20th will mark a year and a half since my diagnosis. Eighteen months of fighting this disease, and so far winning. The Lord supplies me with the emotional and physical strength to do so, and I know through Him, beating cancer is possible.

All my Love,
Christine

through him, all things are possible!

FEB. 21, 2016

Another round down, and three more to go before my next scan. I had a CT scan on February 12th, as I had not had one since November. The results showed that the cancer still grew while I was on chemo-lite, and apparently, it wasn't strong enough to keep it from growing, let alone cause it to shrink. My CEA level went from 1.6 to 4.6. So, my doctor put me back on full-dose rounds to start shrinking the masses again. It had been over four months since I had had a full-dose, so I was not shocked that there had been growth. I started that day and forgot how much different a full-dose is from a chemo-lite round. By the end of chemo, I really wasn't feeling well and even thought about staying over in Rochester. Between stomach cramps, nausea caused by the horrible taste in my mouth, and a pounding headache, it was a very LONG drive back to Eau Claire. As soon as I got home, I went straight to the couch, and that is where I stayed for three days. I still had an appetite, so I ate pretty much everything in my house. With no energy to go to the store, I was eating some pretty interesting food combinations: pickles, dark chocolate, pepper rings... pretty much anything with a strong flavor.

Monday morning came, and after sleeping most of the weekend and lying on the couch for the rest of it, I felt better. I jumped in the shower and hadn't even put conditioner in my hair before I started to feel faint. I quickly got out of the shower as a wave of nausea came over me. I ended up calling in to work and spent another day sleeping and lying on the couch. After two naps and nine hours of sleep Monday night, I was able to go back to work. I was still a little out of it and wasn't even sure if I was going to be able to make it through my whole shift, but I did. When I took the kids outside, the fresh air helped a lot, and we even tried to make an igloo. The igloo lasted about 2.7 seconds and then was a rubble pile. But did they have fun making it!!!

Each day went better than the last, and by Friday, I was feeling almost 100%. So, the first round back didn't go as well as I had hoped, but I survived it and am ready for my next round this Friday.

Yesterday was my eighteen-month anniversary of Fighting Like A Beast! Wow. A year and a half filled with CT scans, biopsies, and countless doctor's appointments. Through it all, I have received endless support from my family and friends, and I know I wouldn't have been able to make it this far without them. And it keeps on coming. My awesome Aunt Jean, along with some of my other aunts, is organizing a benefit for me. There is no tentative date yet, but she is hoping to have it soon. (See Aunt Jean... I didn't mention any dates or months! :) My aunts are pretty much unstoppable when they have decided to plan something. Haha.

Love you all! If anyone would like to help with the benefit, please let me know. I will give more information when I receive it.

All my Love,
Christine

and in march we wear blue!

MAR. 5, 2016

I'm officially out of my twenties, in age and chemo rounds. Round twenty-nine finished up last weekend, and thankfully, it went a lot better than the last. I made sure to plan ahead so that I could have the best round possible. I wasn't seeing the doctor, so it was just labs and chemo, which doesn't always leave me the most time to eat. I packed some snacks and a sandwich and was super excited to get the room right next to the lounge. With enough food in my belly and normal blood labs, we started round twenty-nine! It went really well, and Sarah and I were headed back to Eau Claire. No nausea this week, but a bit of an icky feeling because of the bad taste in my mouth. I went grocery shopping on the Thursday before to be prepared for the weekend. Chemo Baby Larry gives me cravings just like a pregnant woman, and I pretty much eat constantly while awake. This round's craving was cottage cheese and pickles! YUM!!!! With "mostly" healthy choices, I really didn't feel bad about it. However, I did consume an ENTIRE box of Lucky Charms in less than three days. Love me, my cereal!!!!

Worried about my fatigue, I finally took the plunge and tried acupuncture. We have a family friend, Casey, who has Acupuncture for

Wellness over at the Eastridge Center. He has been trying to get me in since I was diagnosed, but my Eau Claire oncologist was against it. Now that I am in Rochester, Dr. Jessica was all for it. So, I tried it out, and it was awesome! He was able to help with tightness in my neck, shoulders, and back, as well as with the ear pain/pressure I have been having. But the biggest help was my fatigue. When I arrived, I felt a little out of it—not really focused. After a few painless needle pricks and some quiet time with a heating pad, I left feeling great. I was alert and focused. My energy continued all day and into the next week. Mondays are usually a little off for me, as I still feel off from chemo, but last Monday went better than most. So, all in all, it was a good round, and I will be going to my next one this coming Friday.

March is Colon Cancer Awareness Month, and yesterday we wore blue to show our support! Now that Sarah and I have every Friday off, we decided to have a little "sister time" yesterday. We started out with a visit with Grandma, and I finally moved the rest of my boxes out of her basement... only took four months. Haha.

It was around lunchtime when we left, so we went and got some sushi! It was so good, and I couldn't think of a better lunch. With full bellies and the snow about to start, we both crawled into our beds for a nap. Man, I can't believe I used to refuse naps, cause I love them now! We even got a little shopping done and got caught up on one of our favorite shows! Over the last eighteen months, Sarah has always been there for me. She goes to EVERY doctor's appointment I have; she drives me when I can't; she makes me food; she goes out to get me food or medicine when I can't get off the couch. And she does it just because she loves me. She is always understanding and loving. She is my cook, my therapist, my maid, my assistant, my fighting partner... she's my sister! Thank you, "Sarah Lee," for always being there for me through this journey!

All my Love,
Christine

my golden round

MAR. 12, 2016

This round has been named my "Golden Round" because it was my thirtieth round at thirty years old. It started with Sarah having a stomach bug, so she stayed home, and my dad went with me. It was another early start, and we left at 5:30 am. On the way up to get my blood drawn, we were in an elevator. One couple in their eighties got off on the fourth floor, and another couple in their sixties got on. They were heading to ten (chemo floor). They had made a comment about us going to floor ten as well, and we told them we were heading in the same direction. Well, because Dad's "Fight it Like A Beast" shirt was visible, they immediately started asking him questions. You could tell they were nervous and new to the process, and under the assumption that we were headed to ten for Dad. So when they asked if we came here a lot, Dad looked at me and replied, "Yeah, what's this, your 30th round?"

"Yep, it is!"

The lady's jaw hit the floor, and she just stared at me. "But you're so young," she replied. Yep, I get that a lot. She pulled off her husband's cap and showed off his thinning hair. "He's only on round four, and they are only doing six." As we got off the elevator, I told her that they were in the right place. She had mentioned that she had been getting some negative comments from her family about the treatment plan they had gone with. Some of her family thought that they should rely only on changing eating habits like clean eating to help heal the body. I literally stopped in my tracks and turned to face the couple. I told her that I have changed my eating habits, I exercise, and have a whole new positive outlook on life, but there is NO WAY I would stop treatment altogether. I told her that the changes I have made are the reason I have been able to tolerate thirty rounds and still have my hair and the energy to continue to work forty hours a week. You could see her face soften and I smile appear on her face. "I'm glad you told us that." I love when this happens! Just a small conversation changed the attitude of someone who is clearly new to his diagnosis. It was eighteen months ago that I was in the same boat, and it was very overwhelming to hear what I "should do/where I should go." No one giving me this advice was ever in my shoes. All I wanted was to talk to someone who had been where I was. So, to be able to give hope and positive reassurance to someone so new to the process made my day!

My blood levels were all normal... well, except for my glucose. Apparently, the entire box of Lucky Charms I ate the chemo weekend before had some effect on it. But it wasn't high enough to cause any concern. So, on to my doctor's appointment. I hadn't seen my doctor for almost a month, so I was excited to talk with her. We have graduated from handshakes to hugs... we're pretty close. :)

She had a student shadowing her, and when she went over my labs, she had mentioned that she had told her "shadow" that you would never guess I was on chemo, let alone my thirtieth round. I had mentioned to her before that I wanted to write a book, and she was interested in how I was going to portray it. She was so excited about it and was even talking about being able to talk to other cancer fighters about my journey and listening to theirs. I really feel like this is what God wants for my life. It makes me so happy to help others just by sharing my story. She gave me a quick physical because it had been a while, and I passed with flying colors. I have heard a lot about immunotherapy, so I asked her about it.

She said there is a new drug (FDA approved in 2011) that has been very successful in trials and is the drug that "cured" President Carter.

How immunotherapy works is that it reboots your immune system. The reason cancer runs rampant in certain people's bodies is that it turns off their immune system. Cancer basically hides in your body, and your immune system can't fight what it doesn't know is there. This new drug takes away cancer cells' ability to hide, and with an added protein, it fights only the cancer cells. It's your own body fighting the disease instead of using toxins to kill healthy as well as cancerous cells. This is an option that is going to be discussed down the road, not something that we are in a hurry to start. Mayo Rochester actually only gets three spots to run the trials, and they are currently full. Even though the drug is FDA approved, they are still working on how much to give, how long to administer it, and how long its effect lasts.

I am fine with someone else testing it out before I go on it. And my rounds are going better and better each time, so I am in no hurry to change up my treatment plan right now. Don't fix what isn't broken. So we talked more about becoming a peer support specialist, and my doctor thinks it is an awesome idea. We decided to continue full doses, and I went upstairs for round thirty. So we got to our room, and wouldn't you believe it, we were in room thirty! What are the odds? Once again, I brought some food and raided the lounge before I started the round. This must be the key to a great round because I did really well. I had so much energy that I even went to dinner when we got back to Eau Claire. I had trouble sleeping, but even today I feel great. I have the windows open and have even taken some short walks outside. My appetite is very high right now, and we even made homemade chicken noodle soup for lunch. Dad came over this afternoon for soup, and we played a couple of rounds of Speed (the card game). Even though Larry has been a pain and gotten in the way, he has no effect on my energy level or attitude. I am even planning on making cookies tonight! I have still been careful not to overdo it and get plenty of rest, but I just can't believe how different round thirty is from round twenty-eight... taking my steroid really helps, go figure!

I have gone on for quite some time, so I will keep this last part short. We have decided to hold the benefit in September to make sure it isn't rushed, and we have ample time to iron out the details. With this said, anyone who would like to volunteer time, items for baskets, or items for our silent auction, please let me know, and I will pass your info on to one of my aunts. I am overwhelmed with all the support and love that I have been shown, and I am so grateful for the life I have been given. Who knows, maybe I will be done with my book by the benefit! Thank you to everyone!

All my Love,
Christine

motel 6?

APR. 8, 2016

Well, it's been a while since I did an update, so let me get you all up to speed! Two weeks ago, Sarah and I were joined on our biweekly journey to Rochester by my amazing friend, Laura. My doctor is always looking to meet my friends and family, so when Laura offered to come with me, I knew I wasn't the only one who was excited. I had been fighting off a cold and had even gone to the doctor the week before, thinking that I had influenza. They ran every test on me, and no abnormal test results were found. I was sent home after they gave me fluids, but with only the direction that if it got worse, to go see my primary care in Eau Claire. I knew I would be seeing my doctor in Rochester soon, so I just went with it, treating my symptoms with cold medicine.

We arrived in Rochester for my routine chemo appointment, and after seeing my doctor, she decided to cancel my chemo for that week. Not gonna lie... I really wasn't looking forward to having treatment. After telling me her symptoms, she decided I most likely had a sinus and respiratory infection and was in need of antibiotics. Having treatment was only going to prolong the infection, and I probably would have had a pretty crummy week or two. She loaded me up with codeine and amoxicillin and sent us on our way. It was a very short visit, but well worth getting medications to make me feel better. I know I rag on Mayo Eau Claire quite a bit, but I had all the same symptoms when they saw me as when I was in Rochester, and giving antibiotics wouldn't have hurt me even if I didn't need them. I went through another week of feeling like garbage when I could have been well on my way to feeling better if they had only prescribed me the meds I needed. I am grateful for what they have done for me in the past, but I will always continue my care in Rochester. Within twenty-four hours of starting the antibiotics, I felt way better and got to celebrate Easter without Larry! Sorry, bud.

So, another two weeks passed by, and another chemo appointment came around, but this time I would have to drive down on Thursday as they were unable to get my CT scan scheduled on the same day as treatment. Let me take a quick second to give a shout-out to my assistant director at Genesis, Jenny. She is amazing! She not only gave me half the day off on Thursday to go down to Rochester; she was also able to let Sarah out early, too. She has always worked with my appointments as well as working with twenty-two other schedules and does an amazing job! Thank you for always taking the stress out of it for me, and to all the awesome coworkers who have filled in my room while I was gone.

Back to round thirty-one. So, we drove down on Thursday afternoon for blood labs and a CT. We went to our normal floor to find out we were not only on the wrong floor but in the wrong building. They told us about a shortcut in the older part of the hospital, and the elevators took forever! Jokingly, Sarah knocked on one of the elevator doors, and the door opened... creepy! We got in and pressed our floor, and once the doors shut, the elevator started ringing like a phone. We looked at each other, and a voice filled the elevator. "Hello?" I responded as I thought that there might have been something wrong with the elevator. The man's voice asked what I heard as "Twelve-o-six?" but Sarah heard as "Motel 6?"

"Um... this is an elevator." It was all I could think to say.

The doors opened, and we exited the elevator laughing to the nurses' station. The elevator had opened on the wrong floor as well. We decided to take the stairs instead of getting back on the creepy elevator. The scan went well, even though I had to drink the nasty liquid, and we headed to the hotel when it was done, only to discover the pool was closed.

Booooo. After dinner, we pretty much watched *Impractical Jokers* for the rest of the night. It was a very relaxing night filled with LOTS of laughter! We even got to sleep in, as my first appointment wasn't until 9:00 am. Dr. Jessica was going to be able to start her day with our smiling faces!! I wasn't even able to be nervous, like I usually am on scan days, cause everything was running early. She sat down and told us that the scans were really good. She first went over my blood labs, and my cancer marker (CEA) had gone down to 3.9 from 4.7 (anything under three is normal). I am working on getting back to the 1.4 it was before I had my chemo holiday. My glucose is still a little high, but I blame the Christmas Cookies, Conversation Hearts, and my Easter basket. Haha. She showed us the scan, and a lot of the masses in my lungs have shrunk in half, and there are even a few that are no longer visible (she won't let me say disappeared). The one mass on my liver didn't change too much, but it is less defined. And there is no sign of the masses that were previously on my lymph nodes or colon! I could not believe it! It was an amazing scan!!!!!! She has me on another four rounds every two weeks and said that if my awesome response continues, she would be willing to put me back on maintenance. God is awesome! Thank you for all the love, support, and prayers I have received. You are a big part of my fight!

All my Love,
  Christine

just keep swimming, just keep swimming

APR. 24, 2016

One more round toward my main goal of survival is almost complete. Thirty-two rounds in and I feel really good! Now that it's getting warmer and more and more produce is becoming available, I've been able to have more motivation in my clean eating, and it has definitely shown quite a difference. My energy level is a lot higher than even my last round, and I have hardly any symptoms. My sleeping pattern has stayed more regular, with sleeping eight to ten hours at night and only an hour to two-hour nap during the day. Dr. Jessica was speaking at a conference in New York (I know... she's a rock-star!), so I met with her amazing nurse, Allison. She went over my labs, which are all back to normal, including my glucose, which had been higher than normal. The round at the clinic went well, and the weekend has gone really well, and I have a few more hours with Larry until I can de-access and be free again. I was worried about how this round was going to go because it had been a very emotional week.

Last Thursday, I found out that a very dear friend of mine passed away in a boating accident. I spent a lot of last weekend feeling numb and in a state of shock. My appetite was gone, and I just kept busy to get through the day. I knew him all my life, as he was my neighbor for fifteen years and was pretty much like a brother to me. It has been a very emotional and trying time, but remembering all the great memories we shared has really helped. Remember that tomorrow is never promised and to always tell those you love how you feel. Miss you, Kyle!

On a different note, I just found out that the poster is almost done for my benefit and is just getting the last final touches added and finalized. Once the poster is done, we can start taking them to businesses, which is really exciting. I have been told that the planning is going well and coming right along... they are very secretive in this process. Haha. Even my dad has something up his sleeve.

Well, it's a short update this time, but I am so thankful for all your texts and calls this weekend, checking in on me and seeing how I am doing!

All my Love,
Christine

the results are in!

MAY 6, 2016

So chemo was on a Thursday this week instead of the usual Friday. Yesterday, Dad and I drove to Rochester for the normal routine. I had a little trouble with labs as my port was being "positional" which just means that fluids go in fine, but it's difficult to draw blood from it. So instead, they just took my blood from my arm. No biggie here. Next, we went to see the doctor and even got in a little early. The labs that were back were all normal, but there were some that hadn't been checked yet (they all ended up being normal). Next, Dr. Jessica brought up the results of my lung biopsy, which they were testing for a genetic marker that would qualify me for the brand-new drug that she first told me about. The one that people have been "cured" with. Well, my biopsy was six months ago, so I pretty much knew that it had come back that I didn't have the marker. I have never been so happy to be wrong! Turns out, I do have the marker, and I qualify for the new drug. She isn't planning on starting me on this drug soon, but she is keeping it in her back pocket. It is still a fairly new drug, and I have been tolerating the current treatment she wants to continue at least until my next scan (which is on June 3rd).

But that wasn't the only good news she gave me. She had them test an actual cancer cell to see how strong, aggressive it is. The results from this test have shown that my body is extremely effective at killing these cells, and that is why I have been tolerating treatment so well. What do ya know... my body is a cancer-killing machine! This also means that any prognosis that they could give me is now way longer than previously thought. Although, to be fair, their information and research they have most is from a much older crowd. And I have not and will not let someone tell me how long I will live! I am truly in the best place I could be and have the best doctors and nurses taking care of me. I was filled with so much hope and faith after talking with her, and was on to treatment. Round 33 went great, and we even got burgers from Five Guys afterward. It was a beautiful day, so we took the scenic route home and had a nice, relaxing afternoon. I slept really well last night, except that I woke up every hour because of hot flashes, thanks to one of my chemotherapy drugs. Today was cleaning day at daycare, and it is oddly enough, one of my favorite days. I was able to work the entire day with Larry in tow and received some amazing gifts and letters from the parents at the center. Their support and love have made working with their children one of the most rewarding times of my life. I am so grateful to be working at Genesis! This is another short entry, but I am exhausted and ready for some Netflix. Have an amazing weekend!

All my Love,
Christine

change of plans

There was a change of plans when it came to the latest round of chemo. Last Wednesday, I had a low-grade fever (99.8 degrees) and a sore throat. Thinking that it was just allergies, I took some cough medicine and went to bed. When I woke up, the fever was gone, and I went to work. I still had a headache and felt pretty crummy, but I tried to push through. Throughout the morning, I started to feel worse, and by the time we went outside, I knew the fever was back. When I took my temperature, it was already at 101.9 degrees, and I knew I was going to be spending the rest of the afternoon in the emergency room. By the time lunch was served, I was on my way to the ER and was praying it wasn't anything serious.

I was put in a room, and the tests began. I had a blood draw, a urine test, and a chest x-ray. All of which came back normal. I was there for a little over three and half hours and was discharged with instructions to take Tylenol to keep the fever down. Not gonna lie... I am really getting sick of having to go into the ER every time I get a fever just to be told they have no idea why it's happening, and with instructions that are common sense. I know that one of these times it may be something bigger, and I am thankful that it wasn't anything bad, but I know I have to pay $50 to do what I was already planning on. The rest of the weekend was pretty much the same as a chemo weekend. All day on the couch with very little energy, but this time I had little appetite as well. All of Thursday and Friday, I was on Tylenol, and my fever still wasn't coming down very far.

Saturday, I stayed off Tylenol for the whole day so I could see exactly how high my fever was getting. It didn't get above 100.8 degrees, and I was worried it wouldn't go down by Monday. I had heard that you shouldn't use Tylenol when you have a fever because it inhibits your body from fighting whatever it is fighting. So, unless it got higher than 101 degrees, I wasn't going to take some. I never hit 101, so I only took Tylenol before bed. When I woke up this morning, I was fever-free. I was still a little tired, but I felt way better, and my headache was gone. Needless to say, chemo was canceled this week and will resume on June 3 when I have my next CT scan.

I am very excited that this weekend I will be in Kansas for a mini-vacation over Memorial Day weekend. I am also excited that I will get to see my Aunt Jean because she is letting me stay over the night before, because my flight leaves at 5:00 am on Friday. But I am really excited to go over some of the benefit details with her when I get back. I can't believe that it's a little over three months away.

My aunts are going to be visiting and calling businesses around Eau Claire for donations and permission to put up fliers. However, not all of my aunts live in Eau Claire, so they are looking for volunteers to help out. If you would like to help out with the benefit, please let me know so I can pass your info on to my aunts. I am so grateful for the support of my family and friends and completely in awe of this benefit.

I hope you all enjoyed the beautiful weather this weekend!

All my Love,
Christine

ace up my sleeve

I had my latest scan on June 3, and it has shown growth in both my lungs and liver. Also, my blood tests had shown my CEA (cancer marker) went up to 4.7 from 3.9. Not a whole lot of growth, but enough to notice. Since my last treatment, I was approved for a new drug called Panitumumab, and we were keeping it as an "ace in our sleeve" until we needed to use it. With the growth, she believes that the drugs I have been on for the last twenty-two months are no longer as effective. After seeing the results, my doctor has switched me to the new drug. I am no longer on my pump (sorry, Larry), and was immediately started on Panitumumab on Friday. This new drug will not cause any hair loss and only comes with one side effect: skin sensitivity. I will most likely get a rash on the top half of my body and have a very high sensitivity to the sun. She has started me on an antibiotic to help with the rash, as well as a regimen to keep my skin well hydrated and keep the rash at bay. This may sound like a setback, but the new drug I was started on goes into the cancer cells and stops them from growing and multiplying. People have been cured on this drug, and I will take a rash and a summer inside if it means that I will be in remission or better yet...

cured. I trust in God and what he has planned for me. He has put so many wonderful people in my life and gives me strength when I feel weak.

So, the first weekend has come to an end, and I have felt really good. Yesterday, I made a cake for a little girl from the daycare, and it turned out great! She was so excited for her Minnie Mouse cake, and Sarah and I even stayed to celebrate with her and her family. I was pretty tired after a full day, so I did end up taking a four-hour nap on the couch. Today, I felt a little tired and hung out on the couch, but I was able to get a lot of things done here and there and only took a two-hour nap instead. Haha. My doctor said that I will feel pretty good on the new drug and that each round after this one will get better and better, as my first dose was a pretty high dose.

So, it's been an "up and down" type of weekend, but I am very hopeful for the results of this new drug and can't wait to see the results.

All my Love,
    Christine

a rash today... a cure tomorrow?

JUN. 24, 2016

It's been a week since I finished round thirty-five, and I am feeling pretty good. I meet with a nurse practitioner in training, and she went over my labs with me. She was surprised to see I had all normal labs. She gave me a quick physical and was again surprised by my lack of symptoms. It was pretty funny because she kept pushing on my abdomen in the same spot, asking if it hurt. After three attempts, I think she finally believed me.

So before I had said that the one side effect of the new drug, I was put on is skin sensitivity with a rash that affects the top half of my body. Well, about one week after my first round with Pantitumab the rash started. Every day, I have to slather on lots of lotion, hydrocortisone, and sunscreen. My head itches all the time and feels like there is sand in my hair. I have dry patches of skin on my neck, cheeks, and eyelids. I pretty much look like a teenager with acne. Yay (that's sarcasm). I spent the week before my last round contemplating whether this was a symptom I could deal with. I looked up the new symptom online (huge mistake) and was horrified by the images of what this drug can do. There were comments from other patients who found the rash so debilitating that they quit their jobs. They couldn't take the way they looked, and some even took themselves off of it because they couldn't deal with it. I began to feel very overwhelmed because I didn't know how bad my rash was going to get. It had only been a few days, and it was already affecting my life. What if I had to quit my job? What was I going to do? I started to get angry with Dr. Jessica because I couldn't understand how she could put me on a drug that caused this much discomfort. Was it worth it?

Now back to my doctor's appointment. So, after the NP in training finished, she went and got Dr. Jessica. She walked in with a big smile on her face and excitedly announced, "You have the rash!" She is WAY more excited about this rash than I am. Let me explain her excitement. Even though I had the genetic marker for this drug, it didn't mean that it was going to work. Like with any drug, there is always a chance that it wouldn't work. The fact that I have the rash is a sign that the drug IS working in my body. I asked her how bad it was going to get, and she said that usually the first dose is the worst because after that, my body gets used to it, and that I may see some flare-ups here and there, but the rash will calm down over time. With some changes to my skin regimen, the rash is way more tolerable, but I still feel like a cheetah some days. So I keep my final goal of total remission in my mind and fight each day.

All my Love,
    Christine

hitting a smooth patch

JUL. 16, 2016

I have had two treatments since my last journal posting, and both have gone very well... besides the rash. Round thirty-six was on July 1st, and I didn't meet with Dr. Jessica, but I did meet with Allison, who is her nurse. She gave me some more tips about how to soothe my rash, especially on my head, but I have found that aloe works amazingly well at keeping the itching at bay. Looks like I may have to invest in my own aloe plant. I switched back to my natural shampoo and may even try baby shampoo to help with it. It was a very low-key appointment and treatment, hence the reason I didn't add its own entry. Round thirty-seven was yesterday, and I was able to see Dr. Jessica. She is still really excited about the rash (go figure), and I even saw a glimmer of excitement in her eyes when I told her I have also acquired the side effects of sores around my nail beds, as well my hair loss has started coming back. She said that the more symptoms I have the better—it's working. Yeah, yeah, yeah. I wish it would work without them. This was my last round before my CT scan in two weeks; needless to say, I am feeling very anxious for the next appointment. Dr. Jessica gave me the option that if the scans were good that I could go on chemo-lite or I could continue on my current treatments. I told her that regardless of the results, I want to continue with my current treatment. This may sound odd to some of you, but if I stop and go to chemo-lite, my rash will go away, my hair will grow thicker, I will be able to enjoy days in the sun... and then I will eventually have to go back onto full doses, and I will have to start all over again. Apparently, this was the answer she was hoping for as she told me, "Right answer." Haha.

Sarah chimed in with, "Well, we are going to do the scan, and there isn't going to be any cancer left, and we will be done." No this isn't Sarah getting her hopes up, she tells me this before EVERY CT scan. She's my optimistic answer to a negative problem. I know she is the reason that I have been able to not only be positive but stay positive. She is always in my corner, fighting when I can't. Sorry, cancer I bet you didn't expect this tag team! Twisted Sisters taking you out one day at a time.

This round has gone better than the last and way better than the first, which means that my body is now working with the new drug (remember cancer-fighting machine). I was able to get a decent amount of sleep last night, thanks to melatonin, and I have had more energy to be off the couch for bits at a time. I have energy it just doesn't last as long as normal. A nap is in my near future. Due to my clean eating, I have begun to crave healthy foods even during chemo weekends, which is great. It's been a bumpy journey, but it feels like I have hit a smooth patch... for now.

All my Love,
Christine

birthday wishes and scan results

JUL. 31, 2016

D r. Jessica was against having a scan the day before my birthday. She didn't want it to ruin my birthday if it was bad news. I told her that I didn't care, and I didn't want to wait. So Friday, we woke up early and were on the road a little after 5:00 am. And this week, my normal "we" was increased by one, my bestie, Kate.

So Kate, Sarah, and I piled into her car and drove down to Rochester. Our first stop was my CT scan, I went back to get prepped, Kate did some schoolwork, and of course, Sarah slept. When I got back to the CT prep area, I asked, as I always do, "Do I have to drink the oral contrast this time?"

"Nope, just water" she said. Birthday present number one.

For those of you who haven't had to drink it, you're lucky. So, I drank a bottle in ten minutes, and within the next thirty, I was done with the scan. Now onto labs. I couldn't eat before my labs or CT scan, so when I got to oncology, I was forty-five minutes early for my scheduled appointment. I went to the receptionist at the desk and pleaded with her if she could get me in early, and she did!

Birthday present number two! I got in, and since my port was already accessed, I was ready for the lab tech. And then my nurse told me that the lab was running behind, so there was going to be a wait. Well, I only waited five minutes, and then they came in and drew my blood. My port worked beautifully. Usually, they have me move around in order to get it work, turn my head, sing, hum, recline my chair all the way back, etc. But I was in and out and ready for some food. We took Kate to Dunkin' and to our comfy couches spot to eat, seeing as we had two hours before our next appointment. We finished eating, talked about normal, everyday stuff, and Sarah got ready to take her fourth nap of the day when I got a phone call from Mayo. Dr. Jessica was ready for me, and I could come up early. So we packed up our stuff and headed up to the ninth floor. I checked in, and then the waiting started... and then the nerves started. This is the point and time that I get anxious. I'm not nervous during the scan itself, but waiting for Dr. Jessica to see me is when it all sets in. So we get called back to the room, and the nurse takes my blood pressure, which once again will not read, and then she goes to let Dr. Jessica know that I'm ready. So we chit-chat about Kate's baby-on-the-way and name choices and whatnot, and Dr. Jessica walks in. Introductions are made, and before Dr. Jessica can even sit down, she says, "Your scans are excellent." This is one of the many reasons why I love her; she doesn't work up to the results, it's the first thing she tells me. She opens up the scans from that day and the one for two months prior and compares them. All the masses in my lungs have shrunk, and the mass on my liver is starting to break down. There are no masses in any of my lymph nodes or colon. She actually said my colon looks completely normal! So four more rounds have been scheduled, and she even let me get away with having only one round during September because I have the benefit and going to Colorado for my nephew's wedding. My labs are all normal, and my CEA (cancer marker) level went from 4.7 to 3.7. Birthday present number three.

So we talked about other things and how everything has been going, the benefit, and whatnot, and the appointment was over. Kate had told me that it wasn't anything like she had expected. Yeah, we only talk about cancer and chemo for about fifteen minutes, and the rest is laughing and other topics. So we were done with three of the four appointments and headed up to chemo. While we waited for the drugs to come up from pharmacy, Kate and Sarah went to go get food for lunch, and I waited to get hooked up. The girls came back, and I got hooked up, and then I started to get tired. I took a nap and Kate worked on schoolwork, and Sarah worked on her workbook. We usually watch *Ghost Adventures* during chemo, but within the first fifteen minutes, Kate decided it was NOT for her. So, we watched *Daddy's Home* instead. Can't go wrong with Will Farrell and Mark Walberg! Chemo was done by 3:30, and we were all exhausted from the long day. We walked to the elevator, and a man in his fifties came shuffling into the elevator. I knew he had just finished a round like me and was dealing with aftereffects. He takes a look at our shirts and asks me, "Did you kick some ass today?" "Yes, I did, round thirty-eight."

"That-a-girl!" He fist bumped me with a smile on his face. Birthday present number four.

It was so cool to be able to relate to someone else going through this journey. I love being able to talk with people, but it's still hard to know if someone is open to it. So many people are sad and angry and may find my optimism insincere, or they don't understand it. I really treasure the connections I do make with other patients, even if they are only a few sentences long. That's why I am so open to sharing my story and having others share my story. If anyone knows someone going through a journey like mine, and they need someone to talk to, I am always open to sharing my story or meeting them. I am more than grateful for the support system I have, but I know a lot of patients don't have that. When you feel alone or forgotten, that's when the sadness fills your heart, that's when the anger takes over. I am not saying that I have never had a bad day. I just had one last week, but I got a text from a friend, and I told her I was upset, and she was there for me. She didn't grill me about what was going on; she just talked to me, let me know she was there. My support is there, and I thank God for it every day. Birthday present number five.

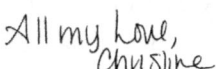
All my Love,
Christine

kicking cancer... not the bucket

AUG. 13, 2016

Well, another round has passed, and I am up to thirty-nine rounds! It's hard to believe sometimes how routine a chemotherapy treatment is. My friend Laura came with me on Friday because Sarah was able to go to the Eau Claire Festival. Thankfully, there were no road closures due to the recent flooding; however, we did end up missing a turn due to us gabbing. Haha. Labs went great, and then it was up to my doctor's appointment with Jessica. First, I saw her NP in training, Akiko, and she did a physical and went over symptoms and labs with me. Last time, my calcium and protein were a little low, but they are back to normal. After I met with Akiko, Jessica came in to go over how I have been doing over the last two weeks. She was really excited that I now have the rash down my legs as well. "The bigger the rash, the better the results." Yep, that's what I keep telling myself. The rash on my head is a lot better now that I have found sprayable hydrocortisone, but I am still having quite a bit of hair loss due to the rash. I know it's due to the rash because my eyebrows have not been this bushy since middle school, and are actually growing back black. So most likely my hair will be black when it grows back. Funny how these things work.

My next chemo appointment is in two weeks, but Jessica was questioning me on why I wanted to cancel the oncology appointment with her. When they gave me my appointment times two weeks ago, Jessica and Allison had no openings on Friday. So they switched it to Thursday. I asked if I canceled my oncology appointment, would I be able to go on Friday just for labs and chemo. This of course worked, so I that's what I did. I think Jessica was a little hurt that I canceled it, but I told her it was the only way they would let me have treatment on Friday. "Oh, I can always get you in for an appointment... you're a VIP." Now I'm sure she tells all her patients that, but I'm not gonna lie, I felt pretty good hearing that from her. So my appointments are all made for August 26th, and I am ready for round forty! Only two more rounds until my next scan. And only one more before my benefit.

After the appointment, we headed up to Gonda 10 for treatment. Laura has gone with me before, but the last time she came, chemo had been canceled because of a sinus and respiratory infection. Not knowing what to expect, she was a trooper! She brought me her AMAZING chocolate chip cookies and gave me an awesome foot rub. I should bring her along more often. :) She had never tried Jamberry before, so we did nails during treatment, and they were pretty awesome. One of the nurses came in and saw us doing nails and gabbing and laughing and asked what we were doing,

"Just kicking it," I replied. Then I thought about what I had just said. "Kicking cancer, not the bucket." She got a good laugh out of it. The rooms that we are given are private rooms that aren't much bigger than a cubicle and lack a door. A curtain can be closed, but I prefer to keep mine open as I am one who likes to connect with people on the same journey. And I was really glad I kept it open yesterday. Across the hall was a patient, not even ten years old, with his mom and dad. And every so often, I would glance in their room and offer a friendly smile when I made eye contact with one of them. As the afternoon progressed, I could see the exhaustion on their faces, the sadness in their eyes, and the defeat in their step. From what I overheard (yes, Grandma I know that it's impolite to eavesdrop, but I felt like I needed to), this was his first treatment, and he even got to go home with Larry! I remember the overwhelming feeling of my first treatment and the numbness that came with it. I really wanted to say something to them, and offer them words of encouragement, but I didn't feel like it was the right time as we were both getting ready to leave.

Laura and I rode the elevator down, and he was all I could talk about, regretting that I didn't say anything before I left. I had to stop at the pharmacy before I left, and God intervened. Who was standing directly in front of us? The boy's mom! The line was long, and I am always hesitant to start talking to people because I know how long and trying those days can be. I made some louder-than-normal comments to Laura as we were in line, "Wow, I can't believe the next round will be forty."

And then it happened... the boy's mom turned around and said, "We're finally at the front of the line."

And that was all I needed. We talked about how long the line was, and then I subtly mentioned that we had been across them during treatment. I had asked if it was his first treatment and where they were from. I found out that it was his first round and that he had been diagnosed only three days prior. They had made the ten-hour drive from Michigan and were planning to do it again in two weeks. I guess my two-hour drive isn't that bad. I had told her that I had started on the same treatment plan that he was on and that they were in the best place they could be right now. She actually smiled and wished me good luck as she was called out of the line. I wish I had given her my information so that I could be an outlet for her. I will definitely be on the lookout for them in two weeks! This has been a long journey, but when I am able to provide someone else with hope, courage, or support it makes it that much more tolerable!

All my Love,
  Christine

2 years of kicking butt!

AUG. 28, 2016

On August 20th, I celebrated my two-year anniversary of Fighting Like A Beast! Sue Ann and her family came up from Chicago for the weekend, and we went for an AMAZING dinner at Mona Lisa's! It was a great, relaxing weekend filled with love and laughter. Friday, I went right back to fighting as I completed my fortieth round of chemo! I ended up not seeing Dr. Jessica this week, as it was a choice between a short day in Rochester or seeing Jessica, which would have doubled the amount of time that we were there. Don't get me wrong, I love my Dr. Jessica, but it was really nice to be able to get back to town before 4:00 pm. Blood tests all showed normal levels, and I have one more round before my next scan on October 7th. Due to my benefit on Sunday, September 11th, Jessica has given me an extra week between rounds, so my next round is on September 16th. So, Friday was a pretty "routine" day and had very little excitement with it. I had trouble sleeping that night, but made up for it last night as I slept fifteen hours! The rash has calmed down on most of my body, but it is still irritating on my legs and scalp. The rash on my head has caused more hair loss than I have ever experienced in the two years of my diagnosis. So hats, scarves, and bandannas have become part of my wardrobe. I'm not sure if it will all eventually fall out, but right now I'm taking it a day at a time.

Right now, I am working on a storyboard that shows the journey that I have been on. As I am putting it together, I can see how many people are on that journey with me. Friends and family who are right there with me, fighting for me when I can't. It is the love and support that I have been shown over the last two years that has fueled my fight!

All my Love,
Christine

Benefit info
Sunday September 11th (2016)
Eagles Club in Lake Hallie, WI 12-5pm

two month recap

I can't believe that it has already been two months since my last update. The last two months have flown by, and I have been so busy, like I'm sure most of you have been as well.

September

At the beginning of September, my mom came down from Kansas and spent the week before my benefit with me. Also, my sister, Jenny, flew down from Colorado for the weekend, so she was able to show her support as well for the benefit. I was completely thrown back by all the love and extreme hard work that went into putting my benefit together and setting it up. It was an amazing and emotional day for me, and I cannot thank you all enough for everything you have done! The benefit was a great success and took off a lot of my financial burden. At the end of the week, I had my forty-first round of chemo. My friend Emily was able to go with me because Sarah had to work, and it was a good round.

Very few symptoms and a good appetite. But that wasn't all that happened during September. I was able to take a legitimate vacation the last week of September to Colorado. My nephew was getting married, and Sarah and I drove down and were able to stay an entire week! It was gorgeous, and we were able to really relax and enjoy the company of our family. It was just what I needed before my next CT scan in October. I was also able to find an amazing wig at one of the shops in Denver, and I am in love with it!

October

October was a little less busy, but not by much. I have started teaching cake decorating classes at Joann's, and I had quite a bit of running around to do after work between the classes, regular errands, and hanging out with friends. I had my forty-second round of chemo on October 14th and had a CT scan as well. The scans showed a little improvement, but otherwise, there was no real change. I had taken quite a bit of time off in between rounds due to the benefit, vacation, and schedule conflicts. The doctor was still happy with the result, as the last time I took some time off from chemo, the masses started to grow back. My blood labs came back normal, so we decided to stay at full-dose and go back to every two weeks. However, this round didn't go as well as the previous ones. I was pretty queasy on the way home and over the weekend, on and off. Monday, I went home from work after only being there for an hour because I was dry heaving in the bathroom (my apologies to the young child outside the door who could hear me. Yuck!). I'm not sure if this was from the chemo or the medication I took earlier, with clearly not enough food. The rest of the week, my appetite was not the best, and I ended up dropping five pounds during it. My appetite slowly came back over the next two weeks, just in time for round number forty-three. We had an in-service at work that Friday, and my co-teacher, Morgan, and I were recognized for our hard work over the last year in our classroom. I was on such a roller coaster in our room before, and we now finally feel like we have a preschool classroom. I was emotional thinking back to how hard and frustrated I was, and so thankful I have an AMAZING management team to help push us to greatness. Love you all, Gayle, Corissa, Jenny, and Jessica! The month wrapped up with our Halloween parade and party. The children all looked adorable and were well behaved for the amount of sugar and excitement that comes with that day. I even dressed up as a giraffe, and the kids thought it was so funny that the teachers dressed up too.

November

The month has just started, so there is not a whole lot of news to pass on. I had round forty-three of chemo yesterday, and so far, so good. My friend Heidi came with me, and I don't think I have laughed that much in a long time. We had a lot to catch up on and were able to enjoy and great lunch as well. Sleeping was a little off last night, but I haven't been able to stay asleep for the last few weeks, so it wasn't too different from before. I am on my last type of herbal sleep aid, Valerian Root, before I have to go on a prescription. Praying it works, unlike melatonin. I am going to try pairing it with yoga before bed and maybe even a sound machine. Any suggestions are welcome! The weather has been gorgeous, and I will hopefully get enough energy to get out and enjoy it before the cold and snow set in.

All my Love,
Christine

happy holidays!

DEC. 17, 2016

Yesterday was a later start than normal. We didn't have to leave until 9:45 am, but with the snowstorm on its way, we left early to get on the road. Get my car all loaded up to hit the road, and my car won't start. Tried it a few more times and nothing! So, we unloaded my car and reloaded Sue Ann's car to get going. The snow had already started, but it lightened and eventually stopped the farther south we went. By the time we reached Rochester, it had started back up a little, but nothing major. The snow caused so many appointment cancelations that we were able to get right in and started a little early even... all good news. No doctor's visit, just labs (which were all great) and treatment. The nurses were very happy with the Christmas Cookies I brought, and I received lots of hugs and thank yous. The nurses on Gonda 10 are absolutely amazing! The things they go through daily are unimaginable, and they always have time for us and have a smile on their face! They know my voice (which is probably because it's so loud) and always ask me about things in my life. Chemo went well, and we even got done a little early. The hospital had initiated an emergency weather plan, and because we were in an inner room, we had no idea how much snow had fallen over the last four hours. We were pleasantly surprised by the actual amount of snow on the ground, as it was still light snow and not a lot had accumulated on the roads. We had to make a pit stop in La Crosse to drop off Christmas Presents for Sue Ann's dad. We weren't able to stay for a long visit as the snow was getting heavier, but we got back on the road and headed home. Sue Ann was driving and strangled the steering wheel the whole way home. We made it home safe and sound, and Sue Ann celebrated with a glass of wine. Haha.

Everything has been going really well, and I have been very busy with Christmas only eight days away!!!! Today, we are finishing Christmas baking with Drops of Heaven and Butter Horns. Some errands will need to be done before our frozen tundra sets back in for the rest of the weekend. Our low tonight is -19 degrees with tomorrow's high at -8 degrees!!! San Diego is looking pretty good right now... think I could talk Dr. Jessica into coming with? It's a good weekend to bake and finish Christmas presents.

I have three weeks off until my next round, and it will be a CT scan as well. Hard to believe it's another year soon, and that in a few months it will mark two years since I transferred my care to Rochester. I only wish I had listened earlier to see an oncologist down there. But in the beginning, I was so scared about the diagnosis that even thinking about switching doctors was so overwhelming. I only dealt with what I had to do that day and could only think about what I had to do the next day. I couldn't think farther than a day into the future without becoming anxious and panicked. Friends and family were not sure how I was taking the news, so in turn, they didn't know how to take it. I started opening up and talking about my fears and concerns with those around me. I started writing down my thoughts and daily events, and my confidence in surviving my diagnosis grew! A fire grew inside me, and I was not going down without a fight. My support team was a huge part of this, and I couldn't have done it without you all!

Happy Holidays!

All my Love,
  Christine

2017

one more to 50!

So, I'm a bit behind from the last round, but here's the breakdown. So last Friday (Feb. 10th), I had my forty-ninth round. Dr. Jessica was not in the office that day, so I met with her nurse Allison, and after talking with her, we decided to up the dose by another 25% from last time (the last round was only 50% because of the reaction I had). So, my dad and I grabbed some lunch and then headed back upstairs for another round. The round went well, and we got back into town a little early.

Because I had a few things going on that weekend, I decided to take my steroids that help with energy. I had a demo on Saturday at Joann's for cake decorating and a baby shower on Sunday. The weekend went really fast, and we still had Valentine's to celebrate. Clay and I celebrated a day early due to conflicting work schedules. It isn't every day I get to come home from work to dinner being made for me, and I don't have to lift a finger! The rest of the week flew by, and by Thursday, I was starting to feel rundown and felt a cold coming on.

By Thursday after work, I could barely talk and now had a low-grade fever. Friday morning came, and nothing really changed. I still had a cough that seemed to come out of nowhere. Then I found out that I had been exposed to influenza A. I immediately got in contact with my doctor and asked her if I should go in and get the test for influenza. She agreed with me, and I immediately went to urgent care. The doctor I saw was awesome and very thorough. He not only ordered an influenza test, but a blood draw and a chest x-ray as well. But he immediately started me on Tamiflu because he said we would be very surprised if it came back negative. My white count was slightly elevated, but not enough to warrant adding antibiotics. So, I picked up my prescription and headed home. I was now under quarantine until I was fever-free for twenty-four hours. Sarah ran to the store for me and grabbed me food for the weekend, and then I sent her away so she didn't get sick. Now I know what you're thinking... Dr. Jessica was upset last time that I didn't have someone with me while I was sick. I talked to Jessica Friday afternoon, and she agreed with me that, with how contagious this was, and as long as I was checking in, she was fine with me being solo. So, I made sure I was eating and staying hydrated. It was a gorgeous weekend here, and every day was sunny and in the '50s and '60s. Can I pick a weekend to get sick or what? Well, my immune system must be working fairly well because my fever broke last night, and I weathered the storm pretty well.

Today, I am still feeling pretty weak and am waiting for the rest of my twenty-four hours to be up when I can actually be around people again. Chemo was canceled for this coming Friday, and my next appointment will be March 10th, when I have my next scan and my fiftieth round! So for the next three weeks, I am trying to get my body back into fighting mode and healthy. Hopefully, I will get to enjoy some of this beautiful weather before the snow takes over again.

All my Love,
Christine

sometimes you just need a beer!

MAR. 11, 2017

So if figured I should get this journal entry up ASAP, as I have been getting lots of texts about how my scans went yesterday. Sarah and I left at 4:30 am yesterday to get down to Rochester. We usually go down the night before when there are scans, but my cat has been sick with a UTI, and I didn't want to leave him alone that long. So, we got down there early for once and did blood labs and my CT scan. We grabbed some breakfast and headed up to the doctor's office. Now I had been nervous for a week or two over the scans, and I have come to find out that I had every right to be. The scans came back showing growth. Jessica says that it's "a little growth," but I decided I didn't want to see the scans. I had already felt discouraged, and looking at them wasn't going to help. Since my last scan on January 6th, I have only had one full-dose. The last two months have been pretty crappy, if I do say so myself. I have been hospitalized for chemo-related side effects, including high fever, dehydration, mouth sores, and a flare-up of my rash on my face. I had influenza and have spent the last two weeks just feeling like crap. My other two rounds of chemo were a 50% dose and a 75% dose. Jessica decided that the side effects aren't worth the results we are getting with this drug. She believes that my body is mentally and physically stressed from chemo, and that it is time to give my body a break, and I 100% agree with her. Sometimes, I think she can read my mind. I haven't had a chemo break for over sixteen months, and boy, do I need one. So, for the next three months, I will be on chemo-lite. This time, it is a pill form that I am on for two weeks of the month. I will also be taking Avastin again and will need to go to Rochester every two weeks for that, as well as doctor visits and labs.

Now that was the bad news... here's the good news! The new drug regimen comes with no side effects! No more rash, no more hair loss, no more sun sensitivity, no more mouth sores, no more super dry skin, no more sores on my fingers, no more cracked fingertips and fingers, no more headaches, no more digestive issues, no more nausea, no more antibiotics, no more steroids, and no more fatigue! Nothing! I will have three months to let my body heal and for me to get it back to fighting status! Yes, it is very discouraging to hear that the cancer has grown, but my body is clearly showing that it is too tired to fight! I am going to take these three months and do what I need to do to be the healthiest version of myself for when I go back to fighting in three months. This isn't a setback but more of a timeout between rounds. My mom texted me, "Cancer may have won the round, but the fight is far from over!" Another bonus is that I can once again drink, as it showed no difference whether I drank or not!

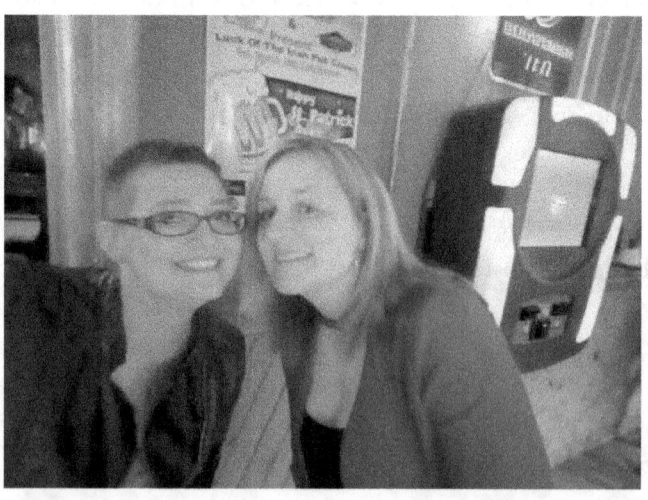

So that's it in a nutshell. Yesterday wasn't a super great day, but I can't control how the scans turned out. I can only control how I react to them. And I choose to eat clean, get some exercise, and relax at the end of a long, hard day with a glass of wine. I choose to spend time with friends and those who are very special to me (especially one in particular). I choose to take a nap when I'm tired and not worry about the laundry I didn't finish. This is the only life we are given, and tomorrow is never promised. Now, if you will excuse me, I'm going to go enjoy a beer!

All my Love,
Christine

me and bert

JUN. 6, 2017

I always feel bad when people ask how I'm doing because they haven't seen a CaringBridge update recently. Honestly, I haven't been posting because I'm pretty boring. Haha. But boring is good in my case. No news is good news, right?

Well, over the last month, I finished my third cycle of Lonsurf. Lonsurf is a maintenance drug that Jessica put me on so I could strengthen my body back to fighting status. It was a nerve-racking three months because I didn't know how or if it was working. And with my hip being injured, I kept freaking out if it was truly an injury or if the cancer was spreading to other parts of my body. No one could give me a definitive action... Do I go to the doctor, or do I rest and ice it? Well, after talking with my team in Rochester, it was decided that an x-ray would be added to my scans that I had last Friday. Nothing like a little bit of anxiety thrown in the mix. So, Friday I had blood tests, a CT scan, an x-ray of my left hip, my doctor's visit, and chemo.

Everything was like clockwork, and after my x-ray, Sarah and I went and got coffee. Lo-and-behold, one of my favorite nurses came into the same coffee shop. Her name is Bert, and she's the best. She even met

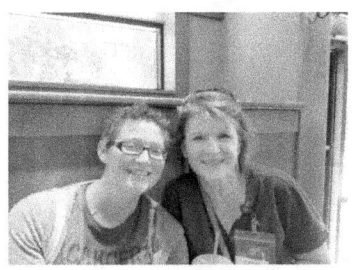

Clay a few weeks ago and totally threw me under the bus. She just kept going on and on about how much I talked about him and that I adored him. C'mon... I mean, who does that? Haha. It took a good five minutes for the red to leave my face. I love her anyway, and even got to take a picture with her.

Sarah and I grabbed some lunch, and while we were eating, I got a call from the doctor that we could come in two hours early. Scans normally take four hours to analyze before your doctor's visit, so going in early meant either really good news or really bad news. Well, we went upstairs and waited. Sarah and I hadn't seen Jessica in about six weeks, and Sarah likes to hide on her. So while we waited for Jessica, Sarah crawled under her desk and waited. Oh, man! She got her good! No worries, I have it all on video, and I will try to upload it to my Facebook.

So once the color reappeared in Jessica's face we went over the results. The new med shrunk all the masses. All we had hoped for was stability, and we were rewarded with shrinking! It was amazing news, and I was so relieved. Because I did so well on the drug she put me on it for another three months. So I will get to go through the whole summer without any side effects! I was over the moon to hear that and so thankful.

Also, last week I became a Great-Aunt... not that I'm bragging about how awesome I am, but that my nephew, Justin, and his wife, Anna, had twin girls, Penelope and Gracyn. They were about three weeks early, but everyone is doing great and already at home! So excited! I can't wait to go see them. So the last week has been an exciting week, but in very good ways! I am so thankful to have so many amazing people around me supporting and cheering me on!

All my Love,
Christine

3 year anniversary

AUG. 19, 2017

Tomorrow is a big day for me. It marks the three years that I have been fighting for my life. Three years ago, today I was diagnosed with stage 4 colon cancer, and it's been one hell of a journey: CT scans, blood draws, ER visits, weekends on the couch, multiple side effects. But through it all, I have received so much love and support from all of you.

I have been taking the chemo drug Lonsurf, which is an oral medication for the last few months with positive results. I started it as a maintenance drug, but it actually started working toward shrinking the masses on my lung. The side effect of the drug, however, is that it lowers my white blood count and makes me more susceptible to getting sick. With working at a child care center, this can be a tricky situation. Well, I succumbed to the stomach flu, as did about one-third of the staff. Because my levels were so low, it took me longer to recover and hit me harder than most. I ended up in the ER with a 105 fever for a blood draw. But this time I made sure to stay hydrated, and took some Tylenol to keep my fever at a reasonable temperature. So, all chemo has been put on hold until September 1st, so I am able to recover completely. On

September 1st, I will also have a CT scan to see the results. Dr. Jessica is hopeful that the results will be positive, seeing as the patients who have seen positive results also have had their white cell counts drop while on it.

I am so very thankful for everyone in my life... all of you, my nurses and doctors, my family and friends. You make it all a bit easier to keep fighting and surviving. I never thought I would have this obstacle in my life, but I have learned so much through it all. Thank you again for your support and love!

All my Love,
Christine

it's not all lollipops and rainbows

SEPT. 3, 2017

Well, August was a very rough month. Four trips to the emergency room, urgent care, follow-ups, stomach flu, and a full-body rash from an allergic reaction. With all that going on, I wasn't able to get back on chemo. I went five weeks without chemo, and it showed in my CT scan on Friday. The cancer ran for five weeks uncontrolled, and the masses in my lungs and liver all grew. But that's not all. The cancer has started to weaken my bones, and because of this, I have a fracture in my left hip. We are not sure when this happened, but the fracture could not be seen two months ago in the last scan. I have had some aches in my hip from time to time, especially when it rains, but I haven't experienced the pain that I would have thought would have come with a fracture in my hip. Because of this fracture, they are afraid that the cancer is moving into the bone and want to start me on radiation. I have an appointment with a radiology oncologist on Thursday to get more information.

As for chemo, I will be going back on the initial treatment of Folfox. This is the medication that gives me neuropathy and cold sensitivity.

And I will be back to having Larry for the weekend (chemo pump). Because I am technically allergic to the med, they want to give me the med a little bit at a time over an extended period of time. I will have to be at the hospital at 6:00 am to start treatment and will be there until about 5:00 pm.

I will have to do this every other week for two months, and then I will have another scan.

The chemo regimen sucks, but it has to be done. I have already done it just not the extended version. But the thought of having to do radiation has completely overwhelmed me. It is an unknown area, and I don't know what to expect.

I'm still in shock and worried about the outcome. I could really use prayers and positive vibes right now. I'm back to living day-to-day and feel like I am back to the beginning after three years.

All my Love,
Christine

ladies and gentlemen, let me introduce... dr. larry

SEPT. 8, 2017

S o, today was my appointment with the radiology oncologist. Sarah and I were back in our old stomping grounds of the cancer center in Eau Claire. My nerves had started to get the best of me the day before, and I wasn't sure what to expect. Sarah and I were given a video to watch about radiation therapy and it answered a lot of questions I already had about it. After the video, the doctor came in. Dr. Larry Past. He even wears a bowtie. It's funny how a name and a bowtie can put someone at ease.

"So, I hear you've been having some pain," he started.

I explained that besides having an achy hip joint when the weather changes, I don't even notice it. I didn't even know I had a fractured hip until a week ago when I had my scan. He reviewed the scans with me; you can clearly see the break on this scan as well as the last scan. He explained the entire process with me about how radiation therapy would go and then said that because I'm not in pain, he would feel fine in waiting on radiation to see how the bone progresses. I 100% agreed with him and decided that unless the pain worsened in the next two months, we would wait to see what the scans look like in two months after my four rounds of chemo. So no radiation for this girl! Hallelujah!

That wasn't the only good news I received this week. I was pulled into the office and offered the 4K assistant teacher position at my work. I was ecstatic to be able to take on this position. The children I will have in class are the same children I taught at one years old and again at three years old. I am so happy to get to teach them a third time!

August was a pretty crappy month, and September was starting to look like it was going to go the same way. But I kept my faith in God and was lifted up by all of my friends and family. Thank you all for the love, support, and prayers that were given to me, especially those over the last week. It was because of all of you that I was able to keep going forward and continue the fight.

All my Love,
Christine

sorry larry! i'm holding out for ned!

SEPT. 23, 2017

God always has a plan, and I don't know why I make my own. Haha.

Wednesday, I received a call from Dr. Jessica at work because she had something she wanted to discuss with me before she saw me the next day. I had taken a blood test three weeks ago, and the results were in. This wasn't just any blood test; this tested the cancer cells in my blood for markers. These markers sit on cancer cells, and there are some chemo drugs that attach to certain markers. The results came back as me having the same markers as a breast cancer patient. No, I don't have breast cancer, just the same marker. But what this means is that I can use breast cancer chemo meds to fight my cancer. There is a trial that is trying breast cancer chemo meds on colorectal patients. Jessica and my oncologist, Grothey, want to start me on this trial.

My first question is, what are the side effects? Answer: fatigue and a possible reaction during my first infusion. That's it. Then I found out they will pay my travel expenses... sign me up!

Thursday, I drove down to Rochester with my best friend Marissa, who just so happened to be visiting from New York. We met with

Jessica, and she explained the trial once again. After that, I signed the consent form for the trial, and it was faxed to the company. I should know by next week if I am approved, but Jessica says I'm a "shoo-in" for it and a prime candidate. This is very exciting, and I cannot wait to start. Knowing that they could take information from my treatments to help cure other patients, or at least give them another option, is very rewarding. We are all fighting together!

Oh... to explain the title. Obviously, I won't be getting Larry back soon because of the trial, and NED stands for No Evidence of Disease. Lots of prayers that this trial is what I need for remission!

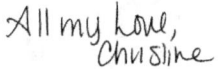

All my Love,
Christine

no one fights alone!

OCT. 7, 2017

Two weeks ago, I was approved to start a trial. The trial is using well-known breast cancer chemotherapy drugs on colorectal cancer patients. After being screened and deemed a prime candidate, it was put into the works for me to start. On Wednesday, I had a new CT scan so the research team can see exactly how much progress this new drug will have. Yesterday (Friday), Sarah and I drove down to Rochester for a blood draw, an ECHO of my heart, and met with Dr. Jessica. She said the ECHO looked great and that we could start the trial that day. Now my nerves have been getting the best of me lately, seeing as this is a brand-new regimen for me, and I didn't know how I was going to react to it. There weren't really a lot of side effects, but my body rarely follows the "normal" path. Because it was my first time and there was a good possibility I was going to have a reaction to one or both of the drugs, they gave it to me over five hours. The first drug took an hour, and then I had to wait for an hour to watch for reactions. Then they started me on the second drug. About halfway through the drug, I started to shake like I was cold, and my teeth started chattering. Soon, my entire body was shaking, and I couldn't stop it. This is the reaction they were waiting for. They stopped the drug and gave me Demerol to stop the shakes.

This is called Rigers [unconfirmed spelling], and they have a drug that counteracts it. So, I was given both and Tylenol to help. After about thirty minutes, they started me back up and I went back to sleeping. I finished the treatment, and they had to monitor me for another sixty minutes. By the time we left the clinic, it was 6:00 pm. Mind you, we arrived at 7:30 am. This was the longest day we have ever had, with driving, we were gone from 5:00 am until 9:00 pm. Yuck!

But one of the nurses explained to me that this is more of an immunotherapy drug, because it only goes after the cancer cells with the specific marker. Hence, the reason I will not lose my hair or have any of the other side effects. It's very exciting and nerve racking at the same time. Now I go back every three weeks, and they will premedicate me before I start, so I won't have to worry about any reactions. Although, they said it usually only happens the first time. The better I do each round, the less time it will take to administer, and soon it will be a two-hour infusion instead of five. Dr. Jessica is extremely hopeful for this treatment to work, and that has definitely helped my nerves.

It's so easy to feel overwhelmed during this journey and to feel all alone. When I was first diagnosed, it was hard because I didn't know a lot of people who had been through it. But over the last three years, I have met so many people who are fighters or survivors or caregivers. We are all in this together... no one FIGHTS alone!

All my Love,
Christine

much to be thankful for!

NOV. 20, 2017

So, I was going to wait until Friday to post, but I received some information today. So far, I have had two rounds on the new trial, and I will be having round three on Friday. With the trial, I have a different schedule for scans and ECHOS. So, my first CT scan was today in Eau Claire. I am not gonna lie... I have been worried about the first scan. I haven't had any side effects, which is nice, but with every other treatment I have always been told that the worse the side effects are, the better it is working. Also, I still have my dairy allergy and have been losing weight when I'm supposed to be gaining weight. So, the thought of having my scan today gave me anxiety, especially when I wasn't going to get the results until Friday! So I went into the clinic, had my scan, and went back to work. Well, within thirty minutes of being back to work, I received a call from Dr. Jessica. I told her of my concerns that the trial wasn't going to work. And then she told me the best news I could have received today. The masses in my lungs have shrunk more after just two rounds than any other treatment she has started me on. I immediately felt better, and a feeling of relief washed over me. I told everyone I saw at work, and I was in such a better mood.

I can't believe how lucky I am that I have no side effects and amazing results. Jessica also reminded me that not only is this amazing for me, but for every other patient who comes after me that they have the research from my trial to cure this nasty disease. It's been a pretty rough week, and this was the light at the end of the tunnel. So as we will be going into the Thanksgiving holiday, I remember just how much I am thankful for.

All my Love,
Christine

not the news i was expecting a week before christmas

DEC. 18, 2017

I have been experiencing headaches on and off for the last two to three weeks. While all last week, it was a constant headache with occasional pressure. I saw Jessica on Friday, and she ordered a head CT, which is in three weeks. Well, I woke up Sunday morning with balance issues and dizziness. Knowing my body, I knew that I had to go into the ER. They did a head CT and discovered swelling and bleeding in my brain, most likely caused by a tumor. So the cancer has moved into my brain. Right now, I am in the ICU being monitored to see if the swelling and bleeding will come down with medication. I have another CT scan in the morning and will know more from there. Right now, it is just wait and see. Thank you for all the love and prayers being sent my way. I am going to need them.

All my Love,
Christine

merry christmas!

DEC. 26, 2017

Wow, what a week! A week ago, I was getting ready to go into surgery; it was only a few hours away. It's so hard to wrap all this around my head, but I clearly needed a step back, and I received it!

I was told that I could leave the hospital after four to five days post-surgery, well that was more like two or three. Home for Christmas was all that I wanted—just to be able to be in my own apartment, surrounded by my friends and family. And after looking at that temperature and wind chill, I was glad to stay bundled up inside. Well, I got the go ahead on Friday morning. I was being discharged, and I could finally go home a mere three days after brain surgery. And then at 8:30 am, I heard the sound I have been waiting over a year for. My ICD was finally ready to be replaced! Yes, this sound was from my chest!

Pause!

Now, I have to wait for cardio to come up. So cardio comes up, and hooks me up. Yep, it's at replacement level, so now I have to get the battery replaced, which originally was gonna last five years, but has lasted seven years. However, this is an outpatient procedure. They cut around the old incision, pop out the old battery, snap in the new, and sew me up. They are checking, but all should be MRI compatible, and I can get MRIs once again. In the grand scheme of things, it's not a big thing to worry about, just something on the to-do list.

Anyway, I'm home with family. My mom leaves tomorrow, and my sister Jenny is coming the 4th of January for a week. Christmas has meant so much to me this year, and I received everything I needed even before the holiday began. Your love and support made the world seem easier, and I am stronger for this fight. I have some consults over the next few weeks, but I am off of everything until I am healed, about four to six weeks. The stitches come out on Thursday after a head CT, just to see what's all going on, and I will have a better idea of when I can get back on this horse!

Staying at home is not my cup of tea. I have already finished multiple crocheting projects, and each day I try to at least get out of the house. Doctor's orders! Everything is going well, and I do have to lay down here and there, but I have to keep reminding myself that I just had brain surgery... which is harder than you think. Haha.

Last but not least... there are a few fundraisers going on that I have been made aware of that were started for me or in my honor. This is very unexpected and always appreciated! The support and love that I have been shown is breathtaking!

1. Facebook Fundraiser - This was started by my sister Jenny on Christmas Eve and has already shown awesome results. All the money raised goes to me (minus a small percent) and will help greatly with bills and food. Being off work for a possibility of six weeks without income does make it a very tense time, but this money will help!

2. Cycle for Survival - This fundraiser was selected in my honor for the Sloan Kettering Research Hospital in New York. The group that has picked me in their honor will cycle for about four hours (I believe), and all money raised will go to the hospital's research.

3. CaringBridge - The funds for this site go to help keep it running. I have never been charged for my three-plus year blogs, and I probably never will! All money donated goes straight back to CaringBridge and gives others the hope, love, and support we all need!

So, thank you! Thank you all again for the well-wishes, the love, the support! Without you, I would have nothing to fight for. Merry Christmas to you all!

All my Love,
    Christine

2018

another surgery down

JAN. 8, 2018

S o, this morning, I had my battery replaced for my ICD/pacer. I have been waiting for two years for the battery to get low enough to be replaced, and among all this, is when it decided it was time to do it. My sister Jenny from Colorado is in town and was able to drive me to and from the hospital. What a way to spend her birthday! It was a pretty standard procedure, and I was in and out in ninety minutes. There is some discomfort where the new battery was put in, but everything is MRI safe! So, the next step will be to meet with oncology and neurosurgery in Rochester.

Today, is the last day to donate to the Facebook fundraiser. Thank you to everyone who has shared, donated, and sent love and light! You are all amazing and I couldn't have done it without you all!

All my Love,
Christine

hope is more than a four-letter word

It has been a long time since I have done a journal entry, and I have been asked many times when I was going to update. I honestly didn't know what to update, as the last six months have been so up in the air. At the end of last year, I found out the cancer had moved to my brain, and I had brain surgery. Then at the end of January, I had radiation on my brain called Gamma Knife Surgery, which wasn't surgery at all, and not at all pleasant. Since the cancer has moved to my brain, all trials have been canceled, and I don't qualify for them anymore. I underwent radiation on my colon and hip at the beginning of March, and that really helped. It was five doses for fifteen minutes. I talked with Dr. Jessica, and we agreed that we would try chemo that I had already been on, but we didn't know what the results would be. I required a blood transfusion as my blood levels were extremely low before I could continue with chemo. I was able to participate in chemo, and it was a very rough two weeks. I was the sickest I had ever been and almost had to be hospitalized.

In April, we took a girls trip to San Diego for a week. It was nice to get out of the snow and into the sun. My numbers had increased, and my energy was better, so I tried another round chemo in May. Once again, I was sick for a week and a half (not nearly as bad), and I was supposed to do it all again in two weeks. During this time, I had a lot of anxiety over chemo and was having insomnia. The weekend before I was to have chemo, I felt horrible, I was achy and sore all the time. I canceled chemo and rescheduled to see Dr. Jessica. I slept like a rock that night. This Tuesday, I saw Dr. Jessica, and together as well as with my mom, we decided that hospice was my best option right now.

My body has fought so hard for the last almost four years that right now it needs to rest. Maybe on hospice for the rest of my life, or until it has time enough to heal, and no one knows this but God. My mom has been great, driving back and forth between here and Kansas, as well as being here for the whole month. Sarah has also been great, helping around the house. She is still working forty hours and takes the time to run errands for me, grab me food, etc.

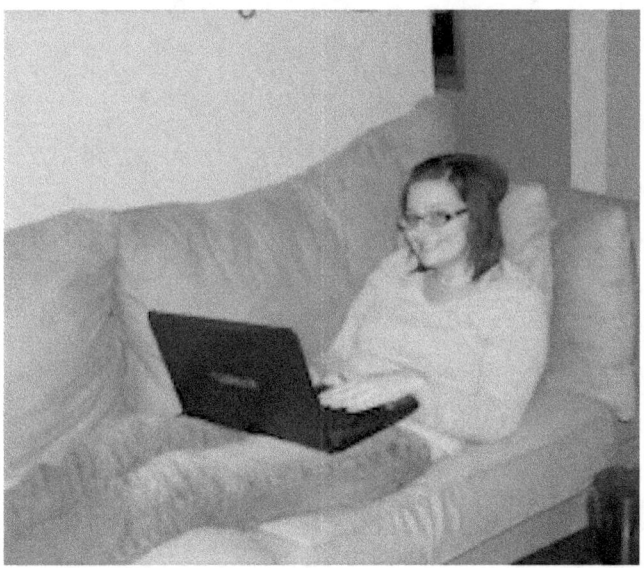

I have just started my hospice intake, so I do not have a lot of infor-mation, but I do know that this is new for everyone and that there have been a lot of questions about my care. Please do not think I am ungrateful for all your support, but I really didn't know what to update. Thank you all for the thoughtful cards and well-wishes. They do make the days easier. Right now, we're just trying to process the information we have been given and get through each day.

All my Love,
   Christine

all my love

JUL. 23, 2018: JOURNAL ENTRY BY SUE ANN COLEMAN

We are mourning the passing of a great soul. On Wednesday night, heaven received an angel. Christine was such a vivacious person with a huge heart and a giving soul. She will be missed and thought of daily. She was the best sister and friend anyone could ask for. She was forever positive and a great warrior in the battle against her cancer, and she fought like a beast until the very end.

Christine was an inspiration. I'm proud to call her my sister. She taught me so many things during her fight with cancer. First and foremost, she taught me what it truly means to be a strong person. She will enter my thoughts daily.

Christine had a motto

Dance like you do when no one's watching.
Love like you've never been hurt.
And...
Live like there's no tomorrow!

We can all learn from this. We can all try to live our lives to the fullest. We can all be warriors in our own way.

We are all warriors in the battle against cancer. This may have been one battle that was unable to be won, but the battle still goes on.

We all must Fight Like A Beast in our own way to help defeat cancer.

Words cannot express the depth at which Christine will be missed.

A visitation will be held from 9:00 am to 11:00 am; a funeral service will be held at 11:00 am with a luncheon to follow. Everything will be at Immaculate Conception in Eau Claire, WI Friday, July 27th.

All Our love,
Janice, Bob, Jenny, Sue Ann, Ken, & Sarah

the fight continues

The end of ones life doesn't mean that the REASON for living can not continue. Christine wanted to help give comfort, hope, and support to those who continue fighting to overcome.

This book was written to fulfill her desire of helping you. Her journey has had that affect on my life, some of the fear has been replaced with *courage*, some of the sadness replaced with *hope* and some of the loneliness replaced with *support*.

As crazy as it sounds... cancer has improved my life.

With *Hope*,
Comfort,
and *Support*,
we can and will get through rough times in our lives.

With all Christine's love for you!

acknowledgments

Thank you Jessica Zalewski for sending the flier "Print to Pro" that started the ball rolling toward publishing; Stacey Smekofske for the editing and taking the vision and making it a reality; Tara Mayberry for the beautiful cover.

A big thank you to Maggie Miller, Christine's dear friend since childhood, who was always a support and sounding board helping her with ideas for the book and for just being there; and Christine's brother, Kenneth (Kenny) Pollack who sadly passed before seeing her book published.

Finally, thank you to Christine's sisters who helped me put this book together and ensured Christine's voice resonated.

about the author

Christine R. Schrader, diagnosed at twenty-nine with colorectal cancer, journaled through her chemotherapy about her relationships and daily life while fighting her fatal disease. She was born into a middle-class family in the Midwest and was the fourth of five siblings. Christine attended Catholic school from kindergarten through her high school years.

She had a well-developed work ethic along with strong managerial and organizational skills. She showed her creative side by making professionally themed cakes. She was able to multitask in the most stressful of times. One of her favorite things was to watch movies starring Keanu Reeves.

in memory of

CHRISTINE REBECCA SCHRADER

Christine Rebecca Schrader, 32, passed away peacefully at home July, 18, 2018, after a four year battle with cancer, surrounded by family.

Born July 30, 1985, in Eau Claire, WI. She is survived by her father, Robert Schrader; mother, Janice (Thesing) Tobisch; sisters, Jennifer (Jeff) Erickson, SueAnn (Kevin) Coleman, Sarah Schrader; brother, Kenneth Pollack; grandmother, Esther Schrader; as well as many aunts, uncles, nephews, nieces, and cousins.

She attended Immaculate Conception Catholic School and was a 2003 graduate from Regis High School. She was working at Genesis Daycare Center until recently. Ms. Christine loved working with children, parents, and faculty. Her smile, organizational skills, creativity, and love she had for children will be remembered by all. She enjoyed cake decorating, crafts, knitting, crocheting, writing, singing, and the outdoors. She had a strong fighting spirit that she used to battle her cancer. For her journey, go to Caringbridge.org to read her story. She will be sadly missed by those who she loved and who loved her.